What did I come in here for again?

How I improved my brain health and memory with the Bredesen Protocol®

To/ Louise
Stay brain fit
Lindsey

Lindsey Byrne

FMCHC,

Certified Re:CODE™ 2.0 Health Coach

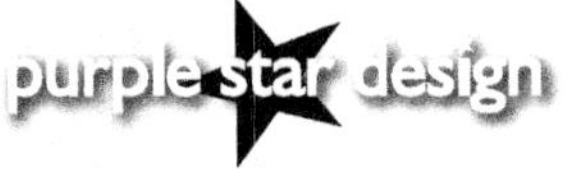

First published in Great Britain 2024 by Purple Star Publishing

Design by Clare McCabe www.purplestardesign.co.uk

ISBN13: 978-1-3999-9036-3

DISCLAIMER

This book should not be used as a substitute for obtaining professional advice and input from a qualified medical professional, Re:CODE™ Practitioner or Functional Medicine Practitioner. The content of this book is generic and while suggestions are made on how to implement good health and wellness protocols, readers are encouraged to contact professionally qualified doctors, Re:CODE™ Practitioners and Functional Medicine specialists to obtain advice specific to their circumstances, genetic predispositions, and biomarkers.

As someone who has always been interested in keeping healthy, especially in terms of healthy eating, I found Lindsey's book insightful. It really displays and explains the links between different aspects of 'being healthy' – many of which are often overlooked – and how this all relates to brain health. I loved the practical exercises and reflective activities which encouraged me to consider aspects of my own health and lifestyle which I had not thought very important before now, in maintaining a healthy brain. I felt like Lindsey was 'holding my hand' and talking with me as I was working through the activities and the coaching sessions, which was very reassuring. I hope this book provides the same reassurance as well as inspiration to others who are looking to improve their brain health and memory.

Lisa

Lindsey has been the consummate professional. She has asked all the right questions and pushed further where it was needed. She is constantly looking for ways to improve things for me, or indeed look for solutions and often goes above and beyond. Lindsey listens and provides a measured response to my questions. She has a positive attitude making exchanges enjoyable and purposeful. Though only with her for a short time I am confident I am heading in the right direction thanks to her.

Richard

This book is a must read for anyone concerned about cognitive health and dementia. It not only shares Lindsey's personal experiences with dementia, but also provides an insightful, comprehensive guide to understanding the factors that contribute to brain health decline. Lindsey outlines the critical steps for tackling dementia and includes self-assessment tools to help readers take proactive measures and take the first steps towards a healthier brain.

Packed with practical advice, invaluable resources and coaching sessions, this book is an essential tool for individuals and families facing the challenges of dementia.

Elaine

An empowering, step-by-step approach that puts you at the heart of your journey and will guide you to create habits and a lifestyle that prioritises your cognitive function now and safeguard it in the future. It's a comprehensive guide packed full of valuable information, tools and motivational tips and a beacon of hope that we can influence our health and wellbeing as we get older.'

Sophia Murray John
Certified Health Coach, FMCHC
Nutritional advisor
Registered Nurse, BA (Hons)
Adult Nursing

Lindsey Byrne weaves her expertise throughout this book supporting you on a self-help journey you can return to time and again. With a previous career in nursing, it was an education for me to learn the importance functional medicine places on discovering and addressing the root cause behind symptoms. This of course makes sense. Should you consider a protocol to prevent or reverse cognitive decline too good to be true, think again. I first heard of the ReCODE™ protocol in 2019 and reached out to Lindsey in 2023 after ill health and surgery led to a further setback in cognition. My memory scores had fallen to 32 when we began working together in the February. On becoming more established on the protocol my memory scores were 92 by the September. Such results speak for themselves. This book is a valuable investment for anyone concerned about cognitive health.

Irene Smith
Author of The A Word, Living in Harmony with My Alzheimer Risk.

The practical content of the book is amazing, it is a text-book,to be referred to on a daily basis. It is truly a practical guide to reducing or reversing the symptoms of cognitive decline.

Alan & Jane

Lindsey Byrne's book, "What Did I Come in Here For Again?" is a powerful testament to the transformative impact of the Bredesen Protocol® on brain health and memory. Through her own journey, as well as poignant stories from her Mum and clients, Lindsey provides a practical manual for those seeking to make positive dietary and lifestyle changes to combat cognitive decline.

This book is a treasure trove of valuable information, offering not only practical advice but also links to further resources, book recommendations, and guidance on sourcing supplements. What sets this book apart is Lindsey's thoughtful approach at the end of each chapter, prompting readers to reflect on key takeaways and take actionable steps towards a healthier brain.

I highly recommend "What Did I Come in Here For Again?" to anyone who values their cognitive well-being or that of a loved one. Lindsey's genuine desire to empower her readers to prevent memory loss and dementia shines through every page, making this book a must-read for those on the path to better brain health.

Allison

This book is for everyone who ever forgot something, walked into a room and wondered why or lost their keys, again and again... and then worried about what it might mean.

This book is intended to bring hope to all, whether you've had parents with dementia or even if you're convinced something is not right, I want you to find the spark of determination to start the fight of your life, so you can look forward to a long, happy, productive life, lived to the fullest.

Contents

Introduction: My story

I'm so pleased that you have bought this book, and I am excited for you to start taking even more control of your own health and wellness and to preserve or even improve your cognitive function.

This book is intended to be my story, to illustrate how the Bredesen Protocol® helped me with my brain health and memory. I will also draw on my Mum's story and a few client stories too. You'll also get access to some of my coaching tools in the appendices, to fit with each chapter in this book, to help you make some changes to your lifestyle should you wish.

I came to Health Coaching after I had been watching my Mum's cognitive health decline for a few years. I saw increasing forgetfulness, some strategies to work around it and some attempts to cover it up. But, like most of the UK population, I thought dementia was a death sentence, that there was nothing to be done. Don't get me wrong, I searched for information, but the first thing I saw on every site was; "age-related, possibly hereditary, no cure". Our family were not the kind to talk about the important things in life and discussion of cognitive function was a definite no-go. So, I pushed it under the carpet and sat back to watch the slow decline.

Mum and Dad had always been proud and fiercely independent, some might say stubborn! They'd always said they would die in their own home. My Dad had been a builder in his career and he'd built their home of 60 years himself when they were first married. I always felt conflicted: I'd always been impressed by their tenacity to keep going and I'm sure it helped them remain relatively fit and independent for so long, despite mine and my brother's worries that whichever of them died first would leave the other unable to cope and our desperate wish to see them settled somewhere safer.

It was early 2019 when my Dad had a health crisis and ended up in hospital leaving my Mum, with her mobility problems, at home on her own. My brother and I were trying to help Mum before and after work, even after Dad returned home during his convalescence, we were so stretched, rushing back and forth, trying to help out. It was such a stressful, difficult time and we realised that we could not allow them to keep living in their large house with a large garden, that they really couldn't cope with, anymore.

I had to sit down and talk to them and point out that this couldn't go on. It sounds ridiculous that an independent woman in her 50's was panicked at the thought of a heart-to-heart conversation with her parents, but maybe you can relate to the strange relationships we can sometimes have with family!

I persuaded them to at least look at the idea of moving to a retirement village and found them a wonderful place, with fabulous amenities and the option of care when needed in the future.

We began the process of moving, we sold their house quickly and started the process of buying their new flat, but before the move could take place, the Covid pandemic struck. The house sale fell through, and everything took a turn for the worse.

We had to try to resell the house in the middle of the pandemic.

My training and coaching business fell apart overnight, my income disappeared and, looking back, I didn't handle that well. With hindsight, I was clearly depressed (not that I would have recognised it at the time) but I was eating rubbish, drinking too much and putting on weight. I started experiencing symptoms associated with menopause; the whole situation was really getting to me. Now I realise, it was actually really fortuitous timing. I would never have had the time to help clear their house and help them move without this break in my career.

We resold the house and Mum and Dad had their health check with the retirement village, which was the first time that we really had Mum's cognitive issues dealt with. They did a MoCA (Montreal Cognitive Assessment) test with Mum. That's a cognitive function test. You might know of it, it's the test where they ask you to draw a clock face, name some animals, list as many words beginning with F as you can think of, give you a name and address to remember, etc. She scored 20/30 which would indicate Mild Cognitive Impairment (MCI). If you've ever seen the MoCA test, I think you'll realise that it's pretty easy to score 30/30 even if you know yourself that your cognition is starting to fail. It's a really blunt instrument. I've heard many stories from clients since, about how their doctor dismissed them after a good MoCA score, saying, "you're fine, there's nothing we can do, come back when you're really getting forgetful".

As soon as the worst of the pandemic restrictions were released, in July 2020, Mum and Dad moved into the retirement village and had to isolate in their flat for two weeks. I deeply regret that. They had no opportunity to explore the village and take part in any activities (they were all paused) and I think this set the tone for the rest of their time in the village. They'd never been particularly outgoing, perhaps they never would have joined in anyway, but my dearest hope was that they'd get involved in more activities and their health would improve a little at least. I now realise that this was my agenda, not theirs. It's taken a while for me to learn that I can't do it all for them.

At this time, I found a little more hope, I pulled myself together and decided to take control of my own health. I started doing the keto diet. I had done it before, successfully, so I knew what to do, but I decided to join a keto diet forum on-line in order to give myself a bit more motivation and find some accountability. It was on this forum that I met someone who was not dieting to lose weight; in fact, he was very slim already. Instead, he was there for support in using the diet to, as he said, "reverse the symptoms of Alzheimer's". Let's just take a pause there. What? "Reverse the symptoms of Alzheimer's"? We just don't hear those words here in the UK! Imagine my surprise! How incredible a coincidence to meet him at the exact right time.

He had two copies of the ApoE4 gene*; predisposing him to Alzheimer's, but more than this, he'd been living with a diagnosis of

*Some people have a particular gene, ApoE4 that raises the risk of getting Alzheimer's Disease. Having the gene by no means guarantees that you will get dementia. People with 2 copies of the gene don't always get dementia. People with no copies can get dementia, but it is seen as a risk factor.)

Alzheimer's Disease for many years and had been forced to leave a high-powered job when he couldn't work around his symptoms any longer, but he appeared completely fine to me! He graciously agreed to chat with me one to one and shared his story about how he had come to reverse the symptoms.

Immediately, I spent the next few days watching countless video clips he recommended from Dr. Dale Bredesen, Dr. Stephen Cunnane and I ordered and read cover to cover the book "The End of Alzheimer's" and then later "The XX Brain" by Dr. Lisa Mosconi.

I was so excited. I searched on-line for practitioners in the UK who could help Mum but couldn't find anyone. I went to the Alzheimer's Society UK to ask, "how can we get a 'cognoscopy™*' for Mum?", but they poo-pooed the whole notion. I didn't give up, I repeatedly asked to talk to their researchers, and eventually I got a response from them that they were aware of the work of Dr. Bredesen, but the trials were too small for them to take notice of. Looking back, I can't understand why they're not funding bigger trials, if the size of the trial is the only issue!

I can't begin to tell you how angry I was. Here was hope. But at every turn it was being denied. Having read, "The End of Alzheimer's" I could see that many people had been turning this dreadful disease around for many years in the US, but I couldn't get anyone to help me here in the UK.

Looking back, I'm horrified at what I did next. I immediately started Mum on some supplements, without having a clue what I was doing. They did make a small difference; she almost immediately seemed a little brighter and started recalling and recounting things from earlier in the week (something that would have been impossible before). But the results weren't as good as I'd hoped. I really don't recommend that approach now. I could have done more damage. Some supplements can be over-done and cause more problems if you take too much or something you don't need.

I eventually found a practitioner I thought could help, but I had doubts that I could get Mum and Dad on the keto diet. Mum's

*cognoscopy is the term Dr. Dale Bredesen uses to describe his in-depth assessment of brain health

mobility was failing, Dad was doing all the cooking and starting to struggle to stand chopping vegetables and preparing the home cooked food they'd always enjoyed and was starting to rely on ready meals. The pair of them were very set in their ways and would find it really difficult to cook and eat a keto diet. Their food preferences were very traditional. The practitioners would only even talk to us if I could guarantee they'd do the keto diet.

I decided that it was my vocation in life to bring Re:CODE™ to the UK, but I wasn't a doctor, there was no way I could train to apply the protocol, but Apollo (Dr. Bredesen's organisation) also trained health coaches, and so my next steps were clear.

Although I was already an executive coach and systems coach (team coaching), I also recognised that working with people on their health was a very different prospect. And I recognised that the way my Mum's physiotherapist talked to her was really skilful and made a big difference to how she looked at her exercises. I had much to learn! I'm sure you will appreciate that working with an executive who has clear business goals or with a team that has a very clear idea of what their problems are, is very different from working with someone with a frightening health diagnosis, particularly when in denial! The challenges increase when it's a family member who can only see you as "her youngest".

It all seemed so serendipitous; I had no work, and so I had the time to retrain. I discovered that I needed to be a qualified health coach already in order to train with Apollo, so after some research I decided to train with the Functional Medicine Coaching Academy (FMCA).

Through them I found a local Functional Medicine Practitioner, who I then discovered had had some training with Dr. Bredesen herself! I was determined to get her to help my Mum, but how to have that conversation... remember in our family, we just don't talk about the important stuff.

I struggled to talk to Mum about her condition, I'm ashamed to say that I tricked her into a GP appointment to assess her cognition in order to open the door to that conversation, but she refused to believe the diagnosis even after seeing a dementia specialist at her GP's practice.

But it did give me the chance to have a conversation and I got Mum to agree to talk to the FM Practitioner. From there on, her cognition started improving steadily.

Mum and Dad still do not even do the whole protocol. Most of the lifestyle changes suggested have not happened. But she took the blood tests and a DNA test and she takes the supplements. She still denies (outwardly) that there is any problem, but on some level, she must realise how much good the supplements are doing. She is still taking them, 3 years on, when normally she is very much against taking "pills" of any kind, despite being an NHS nurse for many years. I credit my upbringing for my own aspirations to live a healthy life without pharmaceuticals whenever I can help it. I wish I could get them to sign up with Apollo; to get the support and community to more fully embrace the protocol, but I think once again, I have to learn that they must make their own decisions.

I started spotting some improvements surprisingly quickly. I initially thought it was just wishful thinking on my part, but then my brother, who had been somewhat sceptical about the protocol, noticed the change.

Then when I took my husband to visit, she asked him for an update on his parsnips (he has an allotment where he grows most of our veggies and some fruits, organically). An unprompted question about something they'd last spoken about three weeks previously. This was a major improvement. Previously, she'd always been aware of what was going on, perfectly able to converse, but unable to remember anything from 15 minutes ago. Furthermore, she'd started to become quite withdrawn, difficult to make conversation with. We watched with such happiness as she joined in playing along with Countdown on the TV, something she hadn't done for months. She became much more engaged and ready to chat.

I was so excited about the improvement; I started to try to talk to people about it. I was so righteously indignant that everyone I spoke to, from the UK Alzheimer's Society, GPs, Dementia specialists and Dementia support workers at my Mum's retirement village were all poo-pooing the idea of any hope of treatment nor even a pause in the decline. This was all despite my experience with my new friend, the evidence of my Mum's improvement and the countless papers and case studies I'd found from others who'd benefited from a Functional Medicine approach and the evidence of my Mum's improvement.

So why the disparity between my experience and the general advice? The scientific process is robust and I am grateful for that. The Alzheimer's Society were very aware of the research I was looking at, but were unable to follow it, as the studies were too small. (Generally, it takes much larger studies and results that are replicated across many studies, to get a drug approved and let's all be grateful for that!) I don't deny that more work needs to be done here too, to test that the results can be replicated.

However, this protocol does not rely on drugs. Most of the protocol is based on lifestyle changes. There are supplements that some people may need to give their body a boost; for example, if they find from blood tests or genetic testing that they are not processing some nutrients well, or not detoxing well, etc. but these are supplements; ie supplementary. At the core of the protocol is the desire to achieve wellness naturally. Many of my clients today find that the side effects of the protocol are other health improvements: pre-diabetes reversing, joint pain clearing up; even my clients' partners often find they're losing weight and feeling more energetic.

Back to my story - Mum was doing well and I had started my FMCA coach training. It all becomes much more personal then, when I discovered through my Mum's testing and treatment that I (in common with Mum) have one copy of a gene that stops me from metabolising B vitamins properly. This leads to a build-up of homocysteine (a natural by-product of eating protein which is normally flushed harmlessly from our bodies) which in turn leads to inflammation – a cause of dementia. Along with the fact that women are twice as likely to suffer from dementia than men, because of hormonal changes that happen in menopause, I'm a little more at risk of dementia than most. I'm just so grateful for discovering FM and being able to put strategies in place now for myself, that will help me avoid dementia later. We only notice dementia symptoms up to 30 years after the damage starts to be done, so, it's never too early to start looking after your cognitive health! At the same time as my discovery, I learned through my FMCA studies, how to better manage my own symptoms associated with menopause and I started to improve dramatically.

Then, one day, my Mum had a fall. She cut her leg really deeply and had to go into hospital. The fall happened at 9pm at night, as she was preparing for bed. She was told to wait for the ambulance, it would be coming soon. They sat up all night and the ambulance arrived at 9am. She was taken to hospital and I thought I'd not be allowed to visit because it was still in the pandemic and restrictions were still in place; my Dad had been in hospital only a few weeks earlier and we'd not been allowed to visit. After a day or two I phoned the hospital to get an update and I was told that as she was on a dementia ward, one person could visit for one hour once a day. So off I went. I was so shocked when I saw her. She was confused, upset, she didn't know why she was there and had no recollection of how she'd got there. This was after just a couple of days without her supplements.

Now of course stopping the supplements wasn't the only problem, apart from that, she'd been awake all night. Now she was in hospital eating terrible food, with no-one to talk to; most of the other patients were very much worse than Mum and some of them were making noise all night, so more nights of poor sleep were on the cards!

By the time we got her home, 17 days later, she was so much worse than I'd ever seen her. It was terrifying! Is this where she would have declined to by now without the supplements? Would we get her back?

The great news is that after just a couple of weeks at home, back in her routine, back on the supplements, she improved so much. She was not quite as good as she was before the hospital stay. But she was able to engage in conversation. She still forgets some things, but often remembers a lot. I'm just happy now if she can stay as she is and halt any further decline. She is completely functional, just a bit forgetful. I've had to re-evaluate my expectations. She's still not making most of the lifestyle changes recommended by the protocol, so this is possibly the best we can hope for.

Today, I'm a qualified health coach, having completed certifications with The Functional Health Coaching Academy (FMCHC) and Apollo Health (Certified ReCODE 2.0 Health Coach) and I'm a ph360 Health Coach as well as completing the University of Derby Bridging the Dementia Divide programme. I'm also member of the UK Health Coaching Association.

I'm the Director of a Health Coaching business: The Cognitive Health Coach, working with clients to prevent, halt the progression of and to even improve the symptoms of dementia.

Since working as a health coach, I have assisted many clients with their whole-body health and wellness issues; brain health is simply an extension of the whole body and cognitive decline can occur for the same underlying reasons and root causes as almost any other chronic illness. My mission is to bring not just cognitive health to my clients, but also to bring a zest for life, a feeling of meaning and purpose. Through improved body and brain health, I am keen for my clients to live fulfilling, healthy lives with the hope and curiosity to truly enjoy their later years.

What brought you to this book?

What was your trigger to say it was time to do something?

I'd love to support you more in your brain health journey, please feel free to contact me here and quote "book" in the comments. https://www.thecognitivehealthcoach.co.uk/contact

How to use this book

It's entirely up to you how you use this book, you may just read it as a story. I hope it inspires you to make some tiny changes to improve your overall health.

If you'd like to go a little deeper, there are self-assessments at the start of many chapters, so you may wish to complete these to assess your baseline before you read the content and tips in each chapter.

Most chapters have a prompt at the end to work through a self-coaching section. Each of these are full of questions for you to ponder, to help you to plan any changes you may want to implement. All the coaching session notes are at the end of the book in appendix 2. If you'd rather not write on the coaching session pages in the book, there are some bonus materials, including these coaching notes available for download on my website.
https://www.thecognitivehealthcoach.co.uk/book-bonus-materials

There's a "wellness 360 map" in chapter 3. You can use this to decide how to prioritise the order you'd like to work through the book. Of course, you can just read it straight through, but if you'd like to pick and choose which topics are most important to you, this will help.

Very occasionally there will be some science and terminology. If you're like me, you'll love all the detailed explanations, but if not, please don't be put off, you don't need to understand the science to apply the lifestyle changes and you certainly don't need to remember any of the jargon. All of the science is referenced to the actual papers, the references are in the back of the book from page 191 onwards

Throughout the book there are links and QR codes pointing you to additional resources and information if you'd like more depth in any of the areas discussed, but they are entirely supplementary, by no means essential; you can ignore them and still get enough guidance to help you improve your brain health and memory.

Chapter 1:

What did I discover that made me think I could change anything?

I'd always believed that we can make a big difference to our health through nutrition. If I wasn't well, I'd always think about what I could do to improve things myself. I'd always had a mistrust of pharmaceuticals. I'd seen so many people start on a drug for a particular ailment, only to suffer side effects, then have to take more and more drugs to counteract those side effects.

We've all probably heard of many home remedies rooted in nature that can help:

- Vitamin C for a cold
- Walnuts for prostate health
- Manuka honey for infections
- Peppermint for an upset stomach

.... just for example.

I don't want to sound like an anti-vaxxer, or to be anti-modern medicine. I am fully up to date on all my vaccinations. For any medical condition, I would always see a doctor and I absolutely encourage you to get medical help for any condition. But what else can we do for ourselves?

I was always disappointed if I asked a doctor, "what can I do; what can I eat (or avoid), what exercises can I do?" and they had nothing for me but drugs.

What has been your experience with the medical profession? Have you wondered if there is more you can do?

Since my studies for functional medicine health coaching started, I've learned so much more about the impact of all elements of lifestyle.

Functional Medicine

Illness is changing. Medicine needs to change with it. We are faced with growing numbers of people living with chronic conditions: Autism, ADHD, Alzheimer's and Dementia, Cancer, Cardio-vascular diseases, Diabetes, Hashimoto's... the list goes on.

> The World Health Organisation (WHO) says; "Chronic diseases are the leading causes of death and disability worldwide. Disease rates from these conditions are accelerating globally, advancing across every region and pervading all socioeconomic classes. The World Health Report 2002: Reducing risks, promoting healthy life, indicates that the mortality, morbidity and disability attributed to the major chronic diseases currently account for almost 60% of all deaths and 43% of the global burden of disease. By 2020 their contribution is expected to rise to 73% of all deaths and 60% of the global burden of disease. Moreover, 79% of the deaths attributed to these diseases occur in the developing countries. Four of the most prominent chronic diseases – cardiovascular diseases (CVD), cancer, chronic obstructive pulmonary disease and type 2 diabetes – are linked by common and preventable biological risk factors, notably high blood pressure, high blood cholesterol and overweight, and by related major behavioural risk factors: unhealthy diet, physical inactivity and tobacco use. Action to prevent these major chronic diseases should focus on controlling these and other key risk factors in a well-integrated manner."[1]

If we all know the risk factors and what we should be doing to avoid chronic disease, what is stopping us? This is where health coaching comes in, examining the root causes of disease and helping clients to find healthier alternatives that suit their needs and are doable

Not so very long ago Type 2 Diabetes was treated as an incurable disease, all that could be done was to treat the symptoms. These days we are all familiar with diets and lifestyle changes that can completely reverse the symptoms of Type 2 Diabetes. It is time to relook at all chronic illnesses through the same lens.

Our current medical practices are well placed to treat acute disease; diagnose, treat with pharmaceuticals, and move on. Chronic illness is different, treating a chronic illness with pharmaceuticals only treats the symptoms; often with drugs that cause side-effects and other imbalances elsewhere in the body.

In fact, the names of many chronic illnesses are not even truly a diagnosis; they're merely a description of symptoms. Alzheimer's for example, according to many specialists, including Dr. Dale Bredesen, is a collection of symptoms caused by many different potential underlying imbalances. To truly treat Alzheimer's and many other chronic illnesses, we need not to look at the symptoms, instead to treat the whole person, to look at any and all imbalances in the body's interconnected systems by looking at:

- Genetic predispositions and risk factors
- Biomarkers to understand how your body's systems are working
- Psychological factors: a sense of meaning and purpose, positivity, stressors in relationships, work and financial matters
- The food we eat and the nutrients we are taking in and how effective our body is at processing them
- The movements we make
- The sleep and relaxation we take
- Our sense of meaning and purpose in life
- The quality of our relationships and connections
- Lifelong learning and brain stimulation

Our healthcare providers (e.g., NHS) are set up to meet, diagnose and treat patients within a very short space of time. For example, a UK patient visiting their primary care provider (General Practitioner) can expect to be allocated a maximum of 10 minutes for their appointment. This is not the GP's fault! This is a function of the (very expensive to administer) healthcare system. GPs are driven to ask closed questions, zero in on the problem, diagnose it very quickly, in order to prescribe a pharmaceutical solution. It's no wonder that they do not have the time to really examine underlying causes and help the patient to find sustainable solutions that will bring long term health and wellness.

Functional Medicine Practitioners can spend a little longer, ask more probing questions, order tests that the NHS can't, optimise (rather than normalise*) the results through a broader prescription of lifestyle changes and supplementation, alongside any necessary pharmaceuticals.

This book is not intended to help you to diagnose or treat any chronic illness, for that you will need to get expert help from a Functional Medicine Practitioner.

Clearly, I'm not suggesting that you abandon your primary care options. Do seek medical advice from all avenues. Functional Medicine Practitioners can work with your primary care team to provide the best and most cost-effective support.

Health Coaching

So, what is the role of a health coach? And why did I decide to retrain as a Functional Medicine Health Coach and Certified Re:CODE™ 2.0 Health Coach?

Have you ever visited your GP or MD and been told to eat more healthily and get more exercise? What exactly did they mean? What changes did they want you to prioritise? How did you implement these changes into your life in a sustainable, enjoyable way?

New clients often tell me that they already eat healthily. Then I

* Have you noticed that when you have tests from the GP, they tell you if you're in the "normal" range? What does that mean? Normal is a statistical term. It means two standard deviations away from the mean. What that actually means is "normal" is 95% of the population. Only the 2.5% at either end of the range get looked at by your GP. I don't know about you, but looking around me at all the obesity, ill health and chronic conditions that are prevalent in our society today, I don't want to be normal. I want to be optimal!

ask them what they eat and they list high sugar, processed foods such as "low fat" fruit yoghurt and granola for breakfast. It's not their fault. It's not easy to pick out what is healthy with all the marketing messages we're bombarded with. I always go by the rule that if the food company has to tell you it's healthy, low fat, high protein, whole grain, etc. on the packet, it probably isn't that healthy! The healthiest foods don't have packaging. Whole foods, veggies, fruits, etc. don't come with barcodes.

Unless you find ways to implement changes that you will enjoy, you are destined to fail, it's not your fault, it is human nature! As Dr. Pat Williams, certified coach, says; "if you could have done it by yourself, you probably would have, by now!"

And that's when I recognised that my purpose in life is to help others apply the Bredesen Protocol®, to get the guidance and support to be able to take control of their own health...

The role of a health coach is to stand beside you as a guide, not to tell you what to do as an expert. We are different from traditional doctors and also different from Functional Medicine Practitioners too. Your practitioner is an expert in their field; a medical professional with additional training in functional medicine, they will recommend lifestyle changes and supplementation to heal the whole of you.

Your health coach will listen to you, really listen. There is no judgement, they will see you as a whole, intelligent, creative person. They will help you to find your own best solutions (alongside the recommendations from your Practitioner) to prioritise, implement and enjoy your new lifestyle. Where it's difficult, they will help you to find workarounds or tiny changes to start the ball rolling.

Your health coach will help you to overcome the sense of "safety" that is holding you where you are now. Even in the midst of a health crisis, we can feel safe or comfortable, doing what we have always done. Your health coach will help you to face growth, no matter where you are right now, to take responsibility for your choices and make the changes you want to see in yourself. We can help you to examine your self-talk, peer norms and find ways to overcome whatever is holding you back.

This book is a story of how I, my Mum and many of my clients have overcome the obstacles to good brain health. Along the way, I'll ask you to reflect on your experience, to help you find your motivation to put the work in. This is not an easy journey; it's the fight of your life, but so worth it. At various points in this book, you'll find a note to some coaching templates at the end of the book for you to work through to help you think through the steps my clients have been through before you.

I had always found the motivation to exercise based on "not becoming my Mum" with her mobility problems. That did work to some extent, but is it really a strong motivator? It just means "not getting as bad as Mum". Even though I might be able to see that I'm better than she was at my age, that still might not be enough. Recently I've become much more specific about what I want to be able to do; I want to ski on my 75th birthday. That is a very long-term goal, but it does mean that I can make shorter tactical goals to support my long-term aim. A negative goal, such as not getting as bad as Mum, losing weight, or some such, gets weaker as you move away from it. If you set a goal to "lose weight" as you are losing the weight, you are moving away from the problem, so losing a bit of weight now, makes the problem seem less urgent. It's easy then for motivation to wane. But if you have a positive long-term aim, then it can only get stronger as you get closer to it.

The first thing I always ask a client is, "what do you want to be able to do, what are you looking forward to?" Many of them talk about seeing their kids or grandkids graduate or marry or meet their as yet unborn offspring. And that's great, there's nothing like a bit of positive thinking; some meaning and purpose in life to keep you going. You've probably all got examples of people you know who "hung on to see their grandkids born" for example. Remember, this is challenging work you're embarking on; how will you keep this sense of purpose at the forefront of your mind when the going gets tough? If you'd like a bit more help thinking through your motivations you can work through the coaching template on page 141 in appendix 2

I'd also like you to think about any successful changes you've made in your life before, whether they were diet, lifestyle or behaviours and habits. What did you do to make them stick? What kept you going? What has worked for you in the past that can work for you again now? Can you find ways to leverage those techniques that were successful for you before, to apply to our work here and now?

Reflection –
What are your key learning points from this chapter?

....

....

....

....

....

....

....

....

....

Chapter 2:
My cognitive health and testing

In addition to some of my symptoms associated with menopause, most obviously, hot flushes and night sweats, I also noticed some minor cognitive changes. I say minor, they're so easy to minimise in your own mind, to explain away or to put down to age or a one-off.

My cognitive symptoms were:

- I would struggle to find a word, quite regularly.

I got adept at working around it, finding a different word, never quite right; not quite sending the message I meant or sometimes I'd just describe the word I was struggling to find.

It's interesting isn't it; I mentioned that my Mum was trying to cover her symptoms? I don't think it's even a conscious thought for lots of us. Whilst there is a stigma associated with cognitive decline, it's completely understandable to cover up, actually I think a lot of the cover up is just a result of trying to "get by".

- I got lost. Twice.

Both times I was quite near home. The first time, I was driving along then I suddenly realised that I didn't recognise anything. I had no idea where I was. I had to pull over and put on my sat nav. I realised in the end that I'd missed a turning and driven straight on, down a road I'd never been down before.

The second time, I was even nearer to home. Again, I was driving along, probably only five minutes away from home and I sort of "came to" and realised that I didn't recognise anything again. Luckily this time, I continued to drive and eventually I came to a roundabout that I did recognise. I realised that I'd actually taken a turning I didn't need to take, I should have driven straight on.

It was bad enough that I'd missed a turning before, but now that I'd actually taken a right turn, that wasn't needed, that really had me questioning myself.

- I was playing Connect 4 with a friend, and I realised I had no idea how to strategize or to win.

This is much worse than it might sound. I am highly competitive and I'd played Connect 4 with this particular friend many times. She's not competitive at all; she doesn't care if she wins or loses and she openly admits that she has no idea how to play the game, really. I'd won against her many times in the past but on this occasion, I lost. Over and over again. While playing I felt completely on the "back foot"; I was playing defensively, with no idea where to put the counters to try to make a line of 4!

If you have read The First Survivors of Alzheimer's – by Dr. Dale Bredesen (it's actually the personal accounts of seven people through the Bredesen Protocol®) you will have read how people dismissed far worse symptoms in the early days. It's so easy to overlook or excuse away these symptoms, particularly when they build up slowly, insidiously. Maybe you'd like to take a moment to think about what you're noticing and consciously assess where you are right now.

Whatever you notice, it could be from symptoms associated with menopause, it could be post-infection inflammation (for example long covid), but it might be the start of something worse.

You might be tempted to put it down to the slowing down we might expect as we age. Whatever the cause, there is much you can do to improve things.

Self-assessment

Symptoms		Not at all	A little	Quite a bit	Extremely
Forgetfulness (e.g., walk into a room and forget why)					
Brain fog (e.g., lose train of thought, difficulty finding words)					
Difficulty focusing (e.g., read same paragraph many times)					
Difficulty learning new things, retaining information					
Difficulty adding up the bill, calculating tips etc.					
Handwriting has deteriorated					
Got lost driving (e.g., momentarily didn't recognise surroundings)					
Depression/lack of motivation (e.g., no longer find joy in hobbies)					
Poor sleep	Trouble getting to sleep				
	Waking in the night				
	Ruminating on thoughts in the night				
Quick to anger					
Slower movements or reactions					
Winter blues (SAD – seasonal affective disorder)					
Can't hear when there's background noise, or tinnitus					
Balance problems (e.g., feeling wobbly, must hold onto stair rail)					
Fatigued					
Flaky nails, white spots on nails, nail fungus					

Cold hands or feet / cramps				
Dry eyes				
Bladder control problems				
Reduced libido				
Bleeding gums				

Risks for poor cognitive health

	Yes	No
A family history of Alzheimer's Disease or another dementia		
Stubborn belly fat		
Brain trauma (accident or sports injury)		
Insulin resistance / pre-diabetes / type II diabetes		
Exposure to toxins or mould (e.g., at work, home or hobbies)		
Mercury amalgam fillings		

Review your answers and make a note of anything that stands out to you, that you'd like to work on.

Where to start?

I decided to take a cognitive assessment. My plan was always to retake the test later to prove to myself that it was working, but if I'm honest it took me a long time to retest. I was a little scared!

My results overall were:	August 2021: **83**	March 2024: . **96**
Made up of: Memory	98	99
Executive Function	55	95
Processing Speed	98	94

So, what does that mean? The test ranked me compared to other people my age and gender. 50 being the average. Whilst I had to be happy with my overall score; I was better than 83% of 53-year-old women, the executive function score was not so good. In addition, there would be a lot of women in the comparison group who were experiencing brain fog during peri-menopause or menopause; 55 was not good enough for me, I needed to take action to improve it!

Before we move on, let me explain the different categories:

Memory is, as you would expect, how well you can remember things. The test shows you various items and then tests you on remembering them, both immediately and also after some distractions.

According to the "Centre on the Developing Child" at Harvard University, "The phrase '**Executive Function**' refers to a set of skills. These skills underlie the capacity to plan ahead and meet goals, display self-control, follow multiple-step directions even when interrupted, and stay focused despite distractions, among others".

Processing Speed can be defined as the time it takes a person to do a mental task. It is related to the speed in which a person can understand and react to the information they receive.

How would you feel about taking this same objective cognitive assessment? This free assessment is comprehensive and granular.

https://www.apollohealthco.com/cognitive-assessment/

Taking this test now, before you start this journey will help you get a base line reading of your cognitive health, and you can retest in a few months to assess how far you've come.

An early client of mine never seemed to get around to doing this cognitive test. I suggested it a couple of times, but I didn't want to "nag"; I should have explored what was stopping him. Anyway, having never taken the test, much later in the process he really regretted this, he had no objective data to provide a comparison. Now I'm much clearer with clients that they will really want to get this done as early as possible so they can enjoy the clear data showing their cognitive health improvements .

What's caused you to think about your cognitive health?... and why now?

Maybe:

- you've noticed some changes in your cognition
- you're noticing some decline in an older relative
- you've had some tests
- you're approaching or experiencing menopause and you recognise that hormone balancing is crucial to cognitive health
- you're just reaching that age where you are keen to make more effort in looking after your health.

Motivation

My motivation was really clear to me. I had always thought that the diseases I most wanted to avoid in life were cancer and Alzheimer's Disease.

As soon as I heard the phrase, "reverse the symptoms of Alzheimer's" it was clear to me that I had to learn more.

I got so excited to think that I could help others to prevent this dreadful disease. I also got really angry that there was so much information available that just wasn't getting to the right people. No-one (it seemed to me) knew about the Bredesen Protocol®, nor about any of the other doctors I've found since, also working on the same principles.

If there's something I've learned in trying to market my services, it's clear that different people need very different motivation.

I genuinely thought that all I'd need to do was talk about what I do, and people would want to know more. Perhaps that was naïve. I also assumed initially that anyone would be prepared to do whatever it takes to prevent Alzheimer's Disease or to improve their brain health and memory. Actually, it's so much more complex than that. We're all busy, we're all supporting other people and probably putting their needs first. We've all been told that there's nothing you can do (even the "miracle" drugs that are currently in the news are only able to slow the decline).

It's the fight of your life. It's not always easy to keep going, when people around you tell you, "it's crazy, there's no cure" or they pressure you to eat badly with an encouraging, "one won't hurt".

If you'd like to explore your motivation and maybe give it a little boost, take a look at the Motivation Coaching Session 1 on page 141 in appendix 2

Testing

Now for the "science bit". Don't worry about any of the technical information coming up in this section, you don't need to remember any of the jargon here.

Mum took the "Full Bredesen Panel" blood test with her Functional Medicine Practitioner. It's available in the UK through a private lab (other labs and other tests are now available - check with your practitioner). It's not quite what it says on the tin. Dr. Dale Bredesen recommends a wide range of testing that may include hormones, gut health, toxins, etc. The "Full Bredesen Panel" is just a blood test, but it does cover a lot of the basics. She also took a DNA test. (As an update, there is now a lab in the UK doing much more comprehensive Bredesen testing).

I took the DNA test at the same time, as a starting point. I later took a homocysteine* blood test and a hormone (DUTCH – Dried Urine Test for Comprehensive Hormones) test too, picking up on my peri-menopause symptoms and a genetic SNP** the Functional Medicine Practitioner spotted. This really helped both me and my Mum to zero in on some actions to take and some supplements that would help us both overcome some imbalances that the practitioner found.

Taking a DNA test can be seen as quite a controversial thing. I was very keen right from the start. Others, I know, are against it. My husband always says he "doesn't want to know". In my view, knowledge is power. The advice for those seeking a gene test used to be, "approach with caution, because if there's nothing you can do to affect the outcome, knowing can only lead to worry".

This is no longer true. We now recognise that genes only create a predisposition (they are the gun) we have a lot of control over our environment and lifestyle. We can change our gene expression through changing our environment and lifestyle (epigenetics***) and unload the gun, or we can pull the trigger if we choose not to make the necessary adjustments.

As an example of this, there is some recent research showing that the indigenous people of the Amazonian tribe of Tsimane carrying 2 copies of the ApoE4 gene[2] maintaining or slightly improving cognitive function! This would imply that it's all about the environment rather than genes.

The ApoE4 gene is considered in the west to increase your lifetime risk of Alzheimer's (from 9% when ApoE4 is negative, to 50-90% with 2 copies)

* Homocysteine is a perfectly normal by-product in the body, produced as we use protein. Most people can easily clear it using B vitamins. I have a fairly common genetic SNP that means I don't methylate (process) B vitamins well so I don't clear homocysteine effectively and a build-up of homocysteine is inflammatory, so now I eat a lot of greens and I take a methyl support supplement.

** A SNP is a Single Nucleotide Polymorphism (pronounced snip). It is not a mutation, it's a very common genetic variation. SNPs represent a difference in a single DNA building block. They can help us to predict response to drugs or to environmental toxins for example. They are not a foregone conclusion, but they can predict some predispositions, that can be altered through lifestyle or supplements.

***epigenetics: environmental changes to make changes to how genes are expressed

Genes are not even the whole picture; a practitioner can test for a multitude of root causes including:

- Hormone imbalance
- Insulin resistance
- Inflammation
- Toxins (be that heavy metals from fillings or seafood, to organic or mycotoxins)
- Your ability to process nutrients
- Brain trauma: an accident or recurrent sporting knocks, for example heading a ball

.... as well as genes.

With so many currently known causes, if you do decide to take some tests, it will be much easier to target specific areas with changes in your lifestyle.

You could find an Apollo practitioner and have a Pre:CODE™ test if you are asymptomatic. Or the Re:CODE™ test if you are noticing some decline in your cognition: https://www.apollohealthco.com

I can thoroughly recommend working with Apollo Health fully; sign up to their programme and you will receive these supportive benefits:

- You can search for practitioners and health coaches in your region or who specialise in your specific causes.
- You'll be able to do a very comprehensive cognitive test (CNS Vital Signs) regularly to see your improvements over time.
- Your practitioner will input all your test results into an easy to read, traffic light report. The report is easy to interpret (link to sample reports over the page) making it easier to interpret your progress if you decide to test and retest in the future.

- You'll also get an app to put on your phone that reminds you when to take your supplements, when to do your brain training, etc. You can add any other prompts you want too, like brush your teeth now, do yoga now, go to bed, etc.
- You'll get access to a monthly "town hall" meeting, where Dr. Bredesen interviews other specialists on topics like oral health, hormones, etc. and answers questions from the audience, so if you need more specific help, you can ask your questions here and get an answer from Dr. Bredesen himself.
- You'll get free access to BrainHQ - the brain training game. To play one game per day is free without registering with Apollo, and you can subscribe separately too. My clients doing the best on the protocol are doing 3-5 games 5-7 days per week. If you are an Apollo client, your practitioner and health coach will be able to see how you're doing with the games.
- You can attend (live or recorded) yoga sessions with an ayurvedic doctor.
- You'll get access to lots of other resources, like KetoFLEX 12/3™ recipes (the diet at the heart of the protocol), etc.
- The opportunity to be part of a community with all the other people who are registered and doing the protocol, to support each other.
- Coming soon to the UK (as is the case in the US) you will be able to get testing and supplement recommendations done before you choose your practitioner, so you can choose a practitioner specialising in your specific issues. You'll also be able to buy supplements formulated specifically for the protocol, saving you money and potentially cutting down the number of supplements you need to take.

* Sample Re:CODE™ Report: https://www.apollohealthco.com/wp-content/uploads/2020/08/Sample-ReCODE-Report-1.pdf

Re:CODE™ stands for **Re**versal of **Co**gnitive **De**cline

Sample Pre:CODE™ Report: https://www.apollohealthco.com/wp-content/uploads/2020/08/Sample-PreCODE-Report-1.pdf

Pre:CODE™ stands for **<u>Pr</u>**evention of **<u>Co</u>**gnitive **<u>De</u>**cline

Whether you need Re:CODE™ or Pre:CODE™ depends on your symptoms. Doing the Cq cognitive test on the Apollo site will lead to a Re:CODE or Pre:CODE recommendation.

It may seem expensive, but compare that to an average month in a dementia care home (more than £2500 in the UK[3])

Alternatively, you could find a Functional Medicine Practitioner https://www.ifm.org/find-a-practitioner/ and discuss taking similar lab tests.

I'd recommend finding an Apollo Re:CODE™ 2.0 Practitioner. Their training will be much more specific. If you're going to do this, do it right. If there's something I've learned from my clients, it's much better to go all in. Take all the tests right up front. Even if you end up implementing the changes slowly, one step at a time, at least you know exactly where you stand. Some of my early clients decided to take the tests a bit at a time. The basics first, treat what was found, then see how far they get, to keep costs to a minimum. The problem with that is that later on, when they have to do more tests, it starts to become tiring. They forget that they'd made that decision knowing it may come to more testing later. Additionally, your causes might be all inter-related. If you don't know all the facts up front, you're just delaying the improvements you could be enjoying. Also, one single blood sample at the beginning is a lot less daunting than knowing you'll be having testing again and again. In addition, of course, there's a cost implication for the blood draws too, so get them all done in one!

Before you decide, write down all your questions for the practitioners here. Review them with a close friend or family member and feel free to go back to each practitioner you speak with more than once, to make sure you're making the right decision for you. You could talk it over with a Health Coach if you've engaged one, they will have a lot more experience of working with different practitioners and will bring more insight to help you to work out what is important to you in finding the right practitioner.

List your questions here:

Once you've taken the tests and had a conversation with your practitioner about the results then you may want to find a Health Coach to help you make any prescribed changes to your environment, food, supplementation, movement, stressors, relationships, etc.

It may seem almost unbelievable that chronic illnesses such as dementia (or indeed cancer, Hashimoto's, ADHD, diabetes, etc.) can be prevented, halted or even, in some cases, reversed with such simple lifestyle changes. However, when we consider how different chronic illness is from acute, and that the causes are almost always an imbalance in our body's systems, it makes perfect sense!

After all, more than 2,000 years ago, Hippocrates, the father of modern medicine, suggested that all disease begins in the gut. Many traditional eastern medicines (Chinese, Ayurvedic, etc.) consider balance between body systems.

Of course, testing is your choice and particularly if you are asymptomatic and simply trying to optimise your overall health and cognitive function, you may choose not to take that route. In that case you can still work through this book, to prioritise what you want to work on.

I'd like to share an example of a client of mine, who did just that, they were able to make just diet and stimulation changes to achieve amazing results:

Case Study:

Here are a couple of case studies of two different people:

The first person organised their own testing with a private phlebotomist, adopted a ketogenic diet and did BrainHQ training for around 30 minutes on average 5 times per week:

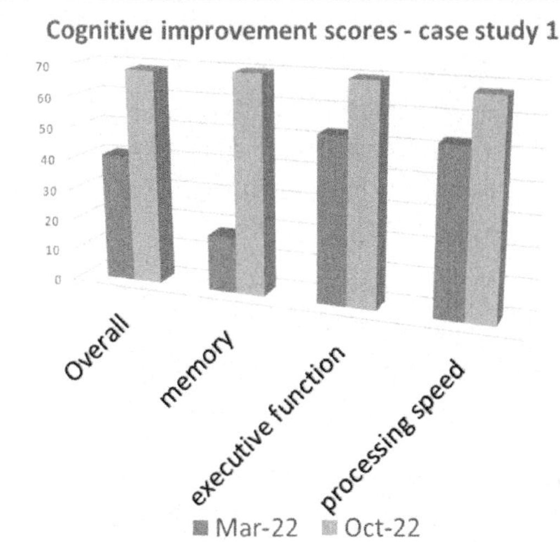

The second did not want to do any testing, adopted a much healthier diet than previously (not ketogenic) and did no brain training, but did dramatically increase her exercise:

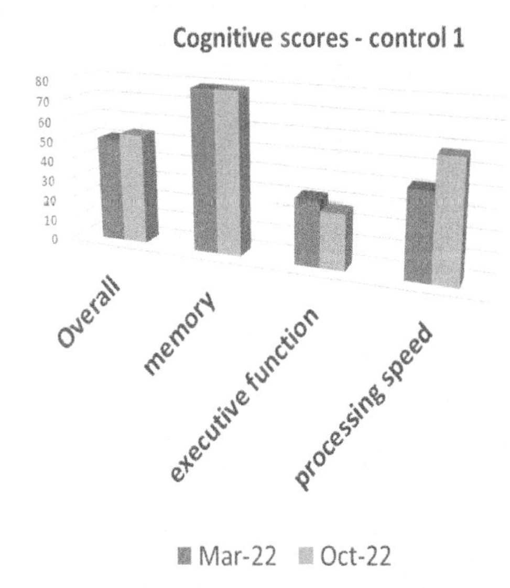

Of course, very little can be concluded from just two examples. What were their comparative health starting points? What contributory factors were each dealing with? These two are amongst a myriad of other questions!

If anything, all that this comparison tells us is that it's a great idea to get tested so you can get a bespoke "prescription" of lifestyle adjustments that you know will have an impact on your contributors to cognitive decline.

Reflection –
What are your key learning points from this chapter?

....

....

....

....

....

....

....

....

....

Chapter 3:

What to prioritise?

I started out prioritising the KetoFLEX 12/3™ diet. It made perfect sense to me; I'd used keto diets in the past to manage my weight. I was used to it. It was easy for me to implement. And now, although all my clients choose their own priorities, unless there is a really good reason to start with something else, we almost always start with the diet. It's such a corner-stone of the whole protocol, why not start there?

My next priority was stress management. I was stressed, it was affecting my hormones. In fact, when I did the DUTCH (dried urine test for comprehensive hormones) I found that my cortisol was rock bottom. That might sound counter-intuitive. Cortisol is the stress hormone. I was expecting it to be really high. In fact, I was so stressed, the FM Practitioner told me I'd all but burned out my adrenal glands! More on this later, in the chapter on stress.

A challenge: Will you commit to prioritising yourself?

As you'll see from this book, although its subtitle is about my health journey, I actually start with a story about my Mum. It's so hard to put yourself first in our society, it's very much expected to help others and put their needs first. That's something that I still have to work hard on in my own health journey.

So, I'm going to start with a challenge! Are you the kind of person who can prioritise their own health and wellbeing? When was the last time you put yourself first? If you'd committed to help someone with something, but you really weren't feeling well, would you invest time in yourself to heal or to rest, or would you feel like you have to stand by your commitment to others?

As they say on the plane, "fix your own mask before helping

others". If you don't prioritise yourself now, how will you be able to help others long term?

This might be your first big hurdle to overcome. Maybe you've been the backbone of the family, looking after the kids as well as supporting your partner, as well as looking after elderly relatives. If you're just not used to investing time in yourself, this is the first step we need to consider.

How can you look at this differently, so that you can prioritise yourself?

Or can you carve out some "me-time" just once a week, to start with, to spend time looking after yourself? When will that be? How will you plan around that? How will you react if others need you in that time?

Now, what exactly will you prioritise?

It's really important that you take control of this whole process. You're the client, it's your journey, you know your body best and you know what's brought you success in the past and what gets in your way.

As a result, we'll be doing assessments throughout the book, for you to reflect on where you are now, what you want to work on, how you will prioritise and what will work for you.

Prioritise your way through this book

This tool is adapted from the Wheel of Life[4], Travis Model[5] and The Bredesen 7[6].

I'd like you to self-score each element according to your satisfaction in each area.

Read through the definitions of each spoke overleaf, to make sure you've considered all aspects of each element.

After you've taken some time to reflect on each, then please mark each spoke from 0 at the centre, to 10 at the rim of the wheel, where 0 is totally dissatisfied and 10 is completely happy, then join the dots to create a plan as in this small example to the bottom right:

Wellness 360° Map

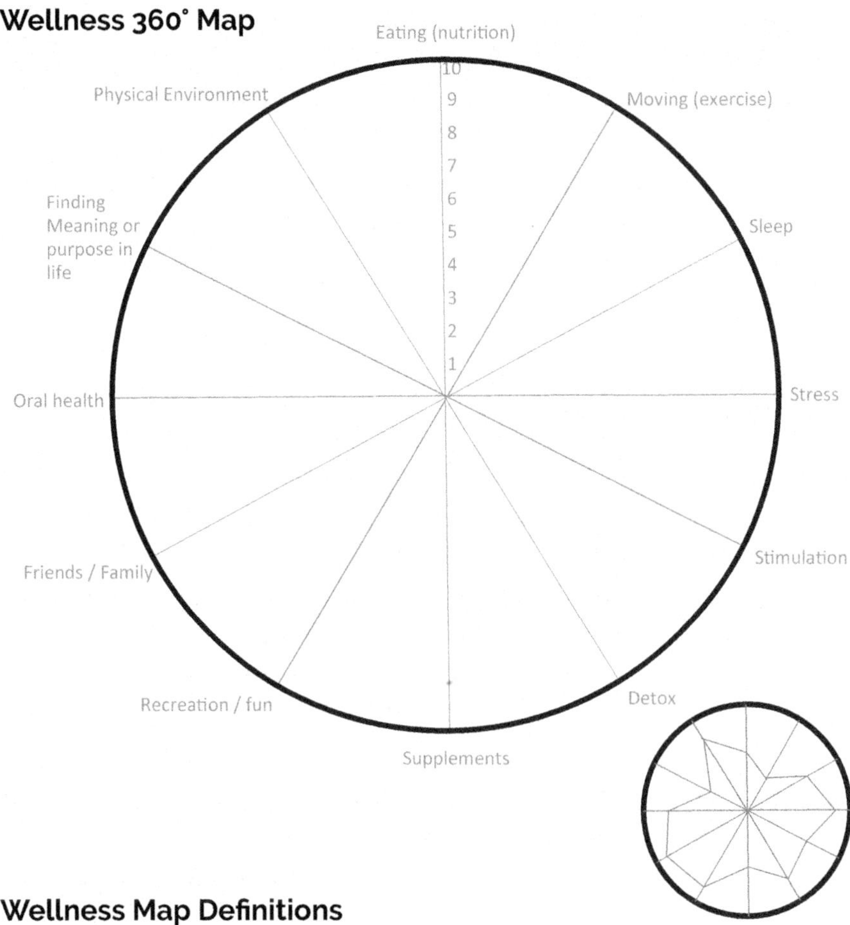

Wellness Map Definitions

Here are some definitions for any of the areas on the wheel that you're struggling to define for yourself:

Eating (nutrition): How happy are you with what, how and when you eat? How do you digest? Does it feel comfortable, happy, relaxed? Is it an enjoyable process of exploration of taste and texture? Or is it something to be rushed, a stressed experience, or leaves you bloated and uncomfortable?

Moving (exercise): How much do you move each day, each hour? Are you taking every opportunity to move to enjoy the feeling, or are you mainly sedentary, or cramming an hour of vigorous exercise into a mainly sedentary day? Or are you in pain, making movement difficult, rather than something to enjoy? Does "exercise" remind you of past, unpleasant experiences for example from school, putting you off the whole idea?

Sleep: How many hours do you sleep, what is the quality of sleep like; do you wake refreshed, or still tired? How regular are your go-to-bed and wake times? How long does it take you to fall asleep, do you wake in the night, how long does it take you to get back to sleep?

Stress: How stressful is your job, your home life, your relationships? Do you often find yourself ruminating on the same problem over and over? How much time do you prioritise for yourself for relaxation? How do you relax?

Stimulation: How do you view learning? What do you enjoy learning? How often do you prioritise learning in your day/week? How curious are you about new things?

Toxins: How toxic is your environment?: In the air you breathe, the things you put on your skin, your homecare products, the food you eat? How comfortable are you that you are detoxing well? Do you sweat? Do you go to the loo every day? Have you been looking after your gut bugs?

Supplements: Have you been advised to take any supplements? Do you take them regularly? How happy are you with the quality of your supplements, the bioavailability (how easily your body can process the supplement) of the ingredients? Are they free of fillers that some manufacturers use, not to aid you, but to make the factory line run more smoothly?

Recreation / Fun: How much fun, recreation and creativity are you enjoying in your work/life balance? How do you prioritise your time for fun?

Family and friends: How are your relationships with others? Is communication smooth and open, or beset by conflict or heartache? How are your closest relationships?

Oral health: Do you have mercury amalgam fillings, do you need root canal treatment, do you have bleeding gums, do you breathe through your mouth at night or in the day, do you wake with a dry mouth, do you dribble in your sleep?

Finding meaning: How clear is your purpose or meaning in life? What spurs you on? What are you looking forward to in life? What's on your "bucket list"? Why not do it now?

Physical Environment: Whether that's your home, your hometown or your work environment; what is it about each of these places that makes you happy, relaxed, content or stressed, dissatisfied or uncomfortable?

It is your choice as to which areas of life you would like to prioritise. Please pick only one or a small number of areas to work on at one time.

If you'd like a little more support as you work through this book, feel free to join my free FaceBook group here: https://www.facebook.com/groups/hopeinalzheimersuk you'll find others in the same situation, who can help with the little things, plus lots of tips, resources, videos and recipes.

Before you start, you might like to take some time to work on a coaching activity to maintain your motivation throughout this journey.

If you'd like to work on your motivation or maintaining it, take a look at the Motivation Coaching Sessions 1 & 2 on pages 141 &145 in appendix 2

Reflection –
What are your key learning points from this chapter?

....

....

....

....

....

....

....

....

....

Chapter 4:

How did I keep this going?

It's a great idea to spend some time thinking about how you've achieved things in the past. You can leverage the same strengths for any new changes that you wish to make.

Something I learned in the FMCA training was how to leverage your strengths to achieve what you want.

I discovered that my signature strengths are:

- Honesty
- Kindness
- Creativity
- Love of learning
- Love

I found it really helpful when thinking about how to keep my desired changes going, to reflect on how these strengths might help me. For example, being honest with myself on what was getting in the way, treating myself with kindness when I slip up and just getting back on the wagon, thinking creatively about nice (non-food) treats for myself when all I can think about is my habit of wanting a glass of wine after a hard day. I love learning new things all the time, so finding out more and more about how food and other lifestyle factors affect our bodies provides even more motivation and in fact, learning is really helpful for keeping the brain active (use it or lose it!) And finally, setting a great example so I can encourage those I love to join me. In fact, there's quite a bit of research to show that if you surround yourself with people you aspire to be like, you are more likely to be successful, whilst people are 57% more likely to be obese if they have an obese close friend[7].

Additionally, I used Tiny Habits®[8] to create some great habits, to remind me to do certain things and to make it really easy not to fail. In his book, Tiny Habits®, B J Fogg PhD, gives us much more information about what helps us to make behavioural changes, over and above simple motivation. New habits must be easy enough (or tiny enough) to overcome the need for great amounts of motivation. Motivation can wane, but if the habit is easy enough, you won't need motivation. We also need a prompt, or a trigger, something to remind us to do the new habit. A great prompt is to tack your new habit onto something that you're already doing habitually at roughly the time you'd like to start your new habit. One of my habits was about exercises. I started with one, "after I walk downstairs in the morning, I will do 1 calf stretch on the bottom step, whoohoo*!

Of course, the idea is that most days you might well do many more, but on your worst days, or your busiest days, you can still do one, so the habit isn't broken. I ended up tacking another exercise on the end of this, and another. Another great example was, as soon as I sit down at my desk in the morning, I will do 1 BrainHQ game. I often do more. I also do DuoLingo (Italian) and sometimes a few other games: wordle, quordle, waffle and blossom. I also have a WhatsApp group where we share our results each day, to help motivate us all to keep it up.

What are the character strengths that you will be using to keep up the good work?

You may well be feeling very motivated at this stage to make some changes. Good for you! Maybe it's all looking like a lot of work, maybe it's feeling a bit overwhelming? That's perfectly understandable and normal!

Research shows us that the motivation to continue and form new habits can come from a very different place from that initial motivation, particularly as you get closer to your goals when you might find it harder to keep going.

* The whoohoo is important (or some other celebration), this small gesture releases dopamine, a neurotransmitter (a bit like a hormone) in the brain that gets us addicted to achievement. It encourages us to keep up the action, so we get more dopamine hits.

This is where calling on your own unique mix of character strengths may help you.

Character strengths are a well-researched, globally recognised area of positive psychology, that can help you to implement and sustain the changes you desire.

There is a free test at: http://LindseyByrne.pro.viasurvey.org and I'd encourage you to take the test and review your report.

Some things to consider:

- The report will list 24 strengths that you hold within you. They are listed by your preference for using those strengths in your life. So, the bottom strengths on the list are not weaknesses, they are simply the strengths that you call on a little less than the others.
- We are likely to achieve more by leveraging our signature strengths (the top 5-7 top strengths listed in the report) than by trying to improve and grow the bottom strengths.
- There will be strengths around the middle of the list, that we are very able to bring forth in particular situations (our phasic strengths)

If you'd like to work on your character strengths or forming habits take a look at the Coaching Sessions 3 & 4 on pages 147 & 149 in appendix 2.

Reflection –
What are your key learning points from this chapter?

....

....

....

....

....

....

....

....

....

Chapter 5:

Food / Nutrition

Even before I discovered the Bredesen Protocol®, I had been using a keto diet for weight management. I did always find that I felt GREAT on keto. My guts felt great (in the early days I was never really poorly outside of keto, I didn't think I was particularly bloated or getting major cramps) but I always felt happy and really calm on keto, plus I did always feel more alert.

My first foray with keto was many years ago on the Atkins diet. That worked for weight loss, briefly, but I never felt like it was very healthy. There were a lot of saturated fats, protein was prioritised and not many veg allowed, so it was only ever a short-term reset for me. I could never keep it up, it wasn't very enjoyable and I was worried about such a reliance on supplements to get all the missing vitamins and minerals. In fact, every time I tried Atkins, it got harder and harder to lose weight. I genuinely put this down to not getting the nutrients I needed, probably because the more I did Atkins, the less I bothered with the supplements. My body was probably crying out for the nutrients needed to live, never mind to process food effectively!

Later on, I found a much healthier keto diet and I discovered that you could eat just healthy fats, but more importantly for me and my views on nutrition, you could eat unlimited non-starchy veg and just a normal amount of protein.

Additionally, Dr. Bredesen's KetoFLEX 12/3™ diet (more on this later in the chapter) includes the idea to "just say no" to inflammatory foods and that includes dairy. I'd always continued to eat dairy on a keto diet; I'd never noticed any lactose intolerance and the DNA test I took didn't show any SNPs for lactose intolerance but eventually, I went through a difficult time and I was suddenly no longer as well as I once had been. I was putting on weight, particularly around my tummy, which I didn't like, but I put it down to peri-menopause... not that I wanted to ignore that. I was working hard to lose weight, but the belly fat wasn't shifting.

Then I started burping, a lot! I ended up with terrible trapped wind and terrible pain. My GP wanted me to take PPIs (Omeprazole) but I wasn't happy about this*, I wanted to look for a more natural approach. I found the iQoro, a simple device that you can use to exercise the muscles around the upper digestive tract, to overcome GERD (Gastroesophageal reflux disease - symptoms burping, acid reflux, heartburn, etc.)

However, at the same time I noticed some scabs on my scalp, then over time they spread to my chest and shoulders! The GP said it was guttate psoriasis, which comes after an upper respiratory tract infection. I had had a bad cold some time before this.

Anyway, I decided that the whole thing: psoriasis, weight gain and burping must be linked and were probably something to do with the peri-menopause, but compounded by stress. I'll say a little more about my stress management in the relevant chapter, but I was also concerned that my microbiome might not be in the best shape after all these pains, so I decided to do some more testing. I was planning to do an elimination diet to see if any particular foods were having an impact, and I took a food sensitivity test (York Test) too. The culprit? Dairy! I'm currently dairy free and improving well.

Menopause and peri-menopause

It's a big concern how much impact menopause can have on all our lifestyle factors. In peri-menopause and menopause three hormones (oestrogen, progesterone and testosterone) start to fall. Oestrogen is very protective of our insulin resistance, stress, inflammation, vascular health and many other areas, so it's no surprise that when oestrogen starts to drop, we might notice changes everywhere in our bodies. It's not so much that these are symptoms of menopause, rather that our stressful lives and some less healthy habits that we used to get away with when oestrogen was providing a protective barrier, are now catching

* I'd read that often acid reflux in older people wasn't too much acid, rather too little, meaning that an oesophageal sphincter is not getting the message to close tight. I'd also read that PPIs damage your microbiome.

up with us. Symptoms of menopause are a wake-up call to start looking after ourselves better. Many women prefer to take hormone replacement therapy (HRT) and given that I'm not a medical professional, I'm not going to comment on that either way, instead I refer you to Dr. Dale Bredesen's "The End of Alzheimer's Programme" and Dr. Lisa Mosconi's "The XX Brain" to find the information you need to make an informed decision on HRT.

Ultra-processed foods

Good food choices are a cornerstone of brain health. The nutrients we get in good quality, healthy food feed our brain. Alternatively, if we eat highly processed food, fast food, food with cheaper ingredients, we are likely to be starving our brains of the nutrients it needs to thrive.

If your food no longer looks like the thing it's made from (ie can you tell it's a chicken or a specific plant) - it's processed. Processing per se is not necessarily evil. Just cooking your chicken simply at home is processing! Cheese is processed milk, but if it's ultra-processed, if it has ingredients you don't recognise and you wouldn't have in your store cupboard or you cannot even pronounce, then that's ultra-processed.

The YUKA app

I thoroughly recommend the YUKA app. The free version allows you to scan the barcodes of food and personal care products and it will list all the ingredients, colour coding them (red for bad, amber for warning and green for good) but furthermore, it will tell you what each ingredient does to the body. It tells you if some ingredients are:

- endocrine disruptors (which disrupt hormones that our bodies use for signalling and messaging throughout our bodies) so that means, even if we are making enough oestrogen for example, it might not be making it to the oestrogen receptors in all our organs and of course that means our brains too!
- carcinogenic, increasing our risk for cancers
- allergenic, causing inflammation

... all of which will affect our brain health and overall body health.

And the final thing the app does, is list alternative, healthier products you can try. I love this app and I've recommended it to all my friends and clients. Many tell me that they take it shopping every time to help choose the best products on the shelves. I've passed on information and advice about additives and ultra-processed foods to these same friends many times in the past, but it seemed they never took any of it on board. Now they love the app. It seems that all my previous advice to "read the labels" was just too hard. The YUKA app is making it so much easier for everyone.

Although the free version provides all this, I decided to buy the premium version. At the time of writing this book, the app is only £12.99 for a year. What a bargain! The extra functionality you get means that you can search for products so you don't have to have one in front of you to use the barcode. I also just like to fund and help out this great team who are helping us live healthier lives, so much more simply.

I challenge you to get the app and go through your food store cupboard and your bathroom cabinet and see what you find. Given that I was already trying (just through scouring labels) to eliminate as many toxins as possible, I was shocked at some of the ingredients I was finding in common, everyday foods and personal care products. For example, I found carcinogenic ingredients in my toothpaste! Imagine that, why would I put that in my mouth?

There's a bigger purpose at stake here. The more of us who stop buying these terrible, toxic products, the sooner big food and big pharmaceutical/personal care companies will be forced to start making better products for everyone!

What eating plan will you follow?

Whilst I will not be advocating any specific diet for you here, there is evidence to show that as we age, our brain becomes less efficient at using glucose for energy and because of this, many experts recommend a ketogenic diet for brain health, particularly as we age. Our brains will continue to be able to use ketones and fats for energy no matter our age. So, you may wish to consider researching the "keto" diet. There are diet book recommendations listed later in this chapter.

Your self-assessment:

How often in a day do you get really hungry?	
Do you eat only when you're hungry or for other reasons?	
Do you "eat the rainbow every day"? 6 colours: white/cream/beige, yellow, orange, red, green, blue/black/purple	
How do you feel straight after eating, bloated, full, hungry, satisfied, craving something sweet?	
Do you ever get bloating or stomach cramps?	
How often do you feel the need to eat sweet foods after a meal?	
How do you normally react to a diet or restriction?	
What diets have you done in the past that have been successful?	
What diets do you consider to be sustainable in the long term? What features would make a diet sustainable?	
What positive and negative associations do you have with food? (e.g., Mum always fed me xx when I was ill, or celebrations etc.)	
Add anything else you think of here	

Review your answers and make a note of anything that stands out to you, that you'd like to work on.

....

....

....

....

....

....

....

....

What diet will work for me?

There are so many competing diet books on the market, I normally do not affiliate with any single one, we are all unique, and what suits you will not suit me.

And, I'm a health coach, not a nutritionist, so I'm not going to recommend any diets or supplements. It would be, at the very least, completely inappropriate and at worst downright dangerous, to recommend any specific diet or supplements to anyone without knowing a lot more about their health and their needs.

As a health coach, I recognise that you know what is good for you; what foods make you feel good, which foods you don't react well to and I stand by your wisdom; you know what you should be doing. My job is to help you to implement the changes you want to make in the priority order you will find easiest and most sustainable, alongside, of course, any recommendations your Functional Medicine or Apollo Practitioner prescribes.

However, if you're doing this alone, there are a couple of suggestions I'd like to make, if you're interested in hearing more:

Variety in your diet

1. The broader the variety of plant foods we can eat, the better. Plants don't just contain fibre, vitamins and minerals which are essential to health, they also contain a vast array of

phytonutrients that work with our bodies to keep us in tip top condition. The larger the range of plant matter you can eat, the more variety of phytonutrients you are getting.

a. You've heard the adage; "eat the rainbow", because different colours of plants will contain different phytonutrients.

b. Alternately, if we aim to eat 30 different plants a week, we will, by definition, get a good range of phytonutrients. And by plants, I mean teas, herbs, spices, nuts and seeds as well as fruit and vegetables. Hopefully you can see that 30 is not too difficult if you add in all these types of plant. The additional benefit is likely that your food will be much more appetising with all the extra herbs and spices you'll be adding!

c. In his book; "Eat to beat disease", Dr William Li breaks a huge range of plants and foods into their effects on 5 key systems in the body, and recommends that we eat 5 different foods for 5 different systems every 5 days (5x5x5 diet), so he is also recommending a wide range of plant foods.

Whichever of these approaches suit your needs best, as long as you are eating a large enough range of plant food, you are probably making a great start.

Organic Foods

2. In addition to varying your diet, please do consider eating as much organic food as possible. Firstly, it will be free of toxic insecticides and chemical fertilisers, but also, the very tools that plants use to fight infection and insects themselves, help our bodies too. So organic plants that have had a harder life, fighting to survive without man's chemical intervention, will contain more of the phytonutrients we need.

I appreciate that organic food can be more expensive. If you can afford to eat wholly organic, please do. If you need to prioritise, there is a guide at https://www.ewg.org It's updated regularly.

The most toxic plants, known as the dirty dozen, contain the highest levels of insecticides etc., that you should aim to eat from organic sources. The clean 15 are the least toxic plants that you can eat more safely as non-organic versions. Everything else falls in between the two, so buy organic or "traditional" as you desire and as your budget dictates.

A simple guide you can start with right now is that any foods that are particularly thin skinned or delicate (eg berries, salad leaves, etc.) are likely to be heavily sprayed to keep them in the best condition. Anything with a really thick skin (eg avocados) are likely to need less chemical intervention. So, buy organic salad and non-organic avocados, then make your own decisions for anything falling between these extremes, would be my approach.

Diet Books

3. There are plenty of books on the subject of diets for cognitive health. If you'd like to do your own research and decide what diet would suit you, I'd recommend starting with these books:

   a. The End of Alzheimer's Programme. Dr. Dale Bredesen

   b. Genius Kitchen, 100 recipes to make your brain sharp. Max Lugavere

   c. Brain Food. Dr. Lisa Mosconi

   d. The Longevity Diet. Dr. Valter Longo

4. If you are confused about all the conflicting health advice in the media; none of which will suit everyone, consider getting a personalised health assessment at https://ph360.me This is a tool giving you specific advice on diet, exercise, environment, work and relationships based on your genetics, anthropometry (scientific assessment of your body measurements), family history, lifestyle, environment and more. Do consider working with a ph360

Health Coach, the information you'll get access to is vast and can seem overwhelming, but a health coach can help you prioritise to get the "biggest bang for your buck".

KetoFLEX 12/3™

Many experts suggest the keto diet for brain health. For example, according to Dr. Stephen Cunnane, ketones can slow down Alzheimer's:

https://www.youtube.com/watch?v=pR8bHXZKZj8

He says that our brains lose some of their ability to use glucose as an energy source as we age, but we never lose the ability to use ketones and fats as an energy source.

As mentioned earlier, although I'm not going to *recommend* any specific diet here, I do recognise that many of you reading this book are looking to implement the Bredesen Protocol®. A cornerstone of that protocol is the KetoFLEX 12/3™ diet. So, it would be remiss of me not to help with that, if that's your chosen approach.

Here's a great image that will help you (shared with permission from Apollo Health):

KetoFLEX 12/3 Brain Food Pyramid

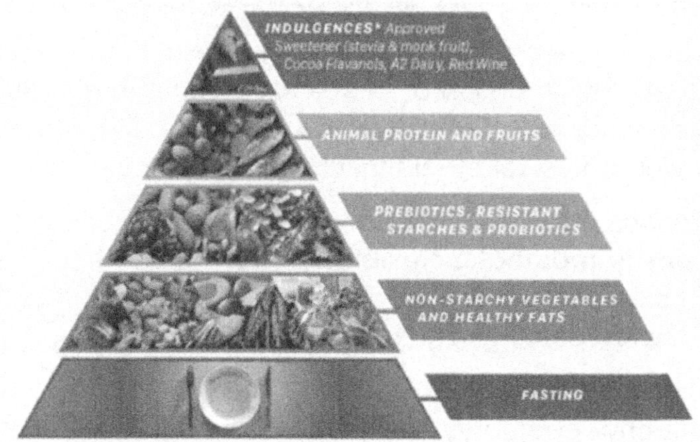

KetoFLEX 12/3 Brain Food Pyramid- BFP © Apollo Health Co

A colour version of this pyramid is available in my bonus content at https://www.thecognitivehealthcoach.co.uk/book-bonus-materials or on the Apollo website.

Keep it Simple

I'd like to make this as simple for you as possible. Lots of advice out there around keto will have you counting macro nutrients (counting your carb grams per day, etc.). I want this to be a lifestyle that is easy to implement, rather than a chore!

(Before I simplify it though, if you are on the Bredesen Re:CODE™ protocol, do take specific advice from your practitioner or nutritionist as there may be specific foods or a specific balance of protein, carbohydrate and fats that would suit you, depending on your test results.)

1. 12/3 simply means:

   a. fasting for 12 hours or more (if you know your ApoE4 status; if you are ApoE4 positive, the advice from Dr. Bredesen is to push that to 14 hours); and

   b. stopping eating 3 hours before bedtime. This can be done overnight. So, if you're eating breakfast at around 8am and finished eating by 7pm, going to bed at 10pm, that's already a 13 hour fast. Easy! But if you're currently fasting for less than 12 hours, build up the fast slowly. Whenever you normally have breakfast, if it's less than 12 hours after your last food of the evening, take breakfast just a little later every day that you feel OK to, until you've achieved your desired fasting window.

   I personally respond really well to time restricting even more than that. My first meal of the day is at lunch time. But that really depends on your health-type. Some people will respond really well to this, for others that might not be suitable.

2. Flex means that you don't have to be in ketosis all the time! **The aim is metabolic flexibility**, that means that you can switch to and from glucose and fat as fuels easily. KetoFLEX 12/3™ involves being in ketosis at least once per day.

3. Start with whatever you normally like to eat. Add more non-starchy vegetables, to fill at least half your plate. Keep your protein to its normal size, do not eat too much protein, too much is not healthy and can knock you out of ketosis. However, it is important to get enough protein, particularly as

we age. If you'd like more specific guidance, take a look at https://www.health.harvard.edu/blog/how-much-protein-do-you-need-every-day-201506188096#:~:text=How%20much%20protein%20do%20I,meet%20your%20basic%20nutritional%20requirements to calculate your specific protein needs each day.

4. Add more fibre (ground flax seeds for example) and healthy fats (extra virgin olive oil, avocado, nuts, seeds, grass-fed organic butter, etc.)
5. Start with foods you love and make small swaps to make the meal keto-friendly.

   a. For example, if you love Spaghetti Bolognese, swap your spaghetti for courgetti (spiralised courgette [zucchini]) and add lots of finely chopped veg to the sauce (for example, onions, carrot, peppers, celery, mushrooms, peas, tomatoes)

You may well have heard of the keto diet as a weight-loss diet. If you don't need to lose weight, you don't have to lose weight with this way of eating. Keto does suppress your appetite somewhat, so we just need to ensure that you are getting good quality, nutrient dense foods. You may lose a few pounds in weight in the first few days, this will be water weight. If you continue to lose weight unnecessarily, make sure you are adding enough healthy fats to your diet. Avocadoes, nuts, seeds and extra-virgin olive oil are very calorie dense. If you continue to lose weight, you might consider carb-cycling.

Carb-cycling

This involves staying in ketosis for a while (say, a couple of weeks) and then eating carbs to increase your calorie intake, (say, for a weekend). Some thought and planning should go into this, are there weekends coming up for you that would suit you to raise your carbohydrate intake. A wedding or a weekend away, for example?

Firstly, it's important to stick to healthy carbs. I'm not recommending going crazy with piles of chocolate cake! Healthy whole grains (for example quinoa, buckwheat, etc.) are good examples. They help you to keep the Glycemic Load (GL*) lower, to stop your blood sugar from spiking, by pairing them with healthy fats (extra virgin olive oil, avocado, nuts or seeds).

Some carbohydrates are more starch resistant. This means they take longer to process in your gut, keep you fuller for longer and feed the good bacteria. You can make some carbs more starch resistant by how you cook them. For example, pasta, cooked, chilled, then reheated is more starch resistant than if only cooked once.

Other starch resistant carbohydrates include:

- Oats (the bigger the cut the better: jumbo oats are better than ones you can microwave). Even better, use just the oat bran.
- Brown rice over white rice
- Beans and legumes
- Cooked and cooled potatoes – eat them cold as part of a salad for example
- Green bananas over yellow bananas
- Quinoa

Finally, how confident are you that you will be able to (will have the willpower to) get back into ketosis? If the temptation to carry on eating carbs will be too much, then maybe carb-cycling is not for you!

* You may have heard of GI: Glycemic Index, which is an index of how much each food raises your blood sugar. GL: Glycemic Load takes into account how much of each food you'd actually eat and how it interacts with other elements contained in that food. GI alone does not tell the full story, because it doesn't account for the many factors that impact your blood sugar. GL represents the quantity and quality of carbohydrates in the overall diet and their interactions in the body. This is why GL is widely regarded as a more reliable tool than the glycemic index alone.

How will you know once you're in ketosis?

Ketosis is the state of using ketones and fats for energy rather than glucose. Once you're in ketosis, you might notice some changes yourself: you might find yourself less hungry between meals, you may lose any cravings you used to experience. If you want to test to make sure you're in ketosis, there are many tools you can use for testing.

Dr. Bredesen recommends that you achieve at least 0.5-4.0 mmol/L of ketones in your blood at some point during the day. You can test this using a breath meter or a blood monitor. If you're an Apollo client, you'll find recommendations for meters to buy and videos to show you how to test in the resources section of your site.

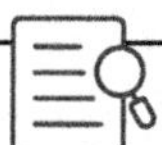

Case study:

One of my clients wanted to test more rigorously than just using urine testing strips, so that she could test different food types, to see what she could eat and stay in ketosis, as prior to working with me her diet had become so restricted, it felt like she couldn't make a "proper meal".

She bought a breath meter as she was planning to test quite a few times over the course of a few weeks, as she tried out different foods. Not wanting to do finger pricks too often, she opted for a breath meter. However, she found she was never in ketosis! So, we tested against the urine strips and got a totally different reading.

Eventually she bought a new breath meter and discovered that the old one had not been working correctly at all!

Do your research, read the reviews of different meters and buy the best within your budget.

Alternatively, you can use a simple urine testing strip.

"Ketostix" urine testing strips are much less accurate, as you're measuring ketones left in urine, after you've used them. If you're using ketones efficiently, you may be using them up and showing only small amounts in your urine. However, if you just want to know if you're in ketosis, any change in colour on the urine strip will show that you have some ketones in the urine, showing that you are in ketosis. Please don't rely on the actual colour change compared to the colour chart on the pack as a measure, as it won't be accurate.

Do I need to test ketones regularly?

If you want to test regularly, that's up to you. Personally, I test to make sure I'm in ketosis as I start the diet. Then I'll only test if I've trialled a new food, to make sure I'm still in ketosis. However, I'm only on the prevention protocol. If you are experiencing symptoms and you're trying to apply the full Re:CODE™ protocol robustly, you will want to be more rigorous and ensure that you're in the right range of ketone production at least once per day.

Different people can tolerate different levels of carbohydrates and stay in ketosis, so you can use the urine test strips or breath meter to find out how much of any given carbohydrate you can tolerate, by trial and error. My recommendation would be to start with only non-starchy, not very sweet vegetables, for example, exclude carrots and peas and exclude fruits. But then, once you're in ketosis, try out different veg and try the least sweet fruits. As you get into the diet, you could try some more fruit. Most people can eat berries and stay in ketosis and blueberries are very good for the brain!

Many people who are very active find they can burn quite a few carbohydrates and stay in ketosis. You might, therefore, want to take your activity level into consideration when deciding the amount of carbs to cut out as you first venture into a ketogenic diet.

Keto Food Swaps

There are many foods you can swap to make your favourite meals or recipes keto-friendly.

Here are some common ones. Add your own ideas to this list:

Non-Keto foods	Swap for these keto-friendly foods
Potatoes	Celeriac, Swede
Rice	Cauliflower rice
Pasta	Courgetti (spiralised courgette) (Zucchini in US)
Bread	There are recipes online and ready to buy keto breads. However, if you just fancy a sandwich or wrap, what about wrapping your fillings in a lettuce leaf or nori sheet?
Add your own ideas here	

Keto-flu

You may have heard of "keto-flu". It's not 'flu! It's a reaction to sugar withdrawal (as your body changes from using glucose as an energy source, to using ketones) coupled with dehydration and mineral loss that can cause some fatigue and/or headaches. This will only happen in the first few days of a ketogenic diet, while you are not yet used to using ketones and fats for energy.

According to Dr. Bredesen, you can overcome "keto-flu" with:

1. Staying properly hydrated - many experts recommend drinking around 2 litres of water per day
2. Replacing the electrolytes lost with water loss - use sea salt

or Himalayan pink salt in your food, these salts contain more minerals than table salt or try an electrolyte mix such as LMNT (That's not an abbreviation, that's the name, pronounced "element").

3. Use MCT* oil or powder while you prepare to start your ketogenic diet. As you are slowly cutting down on your carbohydrate intake, build up using MCT oil or powder, it encourages your liver to start making ketones.

MCT Oil or powder

Many of my clients choose to start using MCT powder before starting the KetoFLEX 12/3™ diet. This can help with the transition to using ketones and fats for energy and stop you ever getting "keto-flu" in the first place.

MCT oil can cause some upset stomachs at first (MCT powder less so), simply because you're not used to it. Start with 1 teaspoon in a coffee and whizz it up with a milk frother/blender, 1 per day. Do this for a few days and only if you still feel fine, then move up to 2 teaspoons, stick with that for a few days, then move up to 1 tablespoon. You can go to 2 tablespoons if you'd like, and maybe spread them over 2 coffees if you prefer. The powder does have the appearance of a creamer, whizzed up in your coffee it does make something similar to a frothy latte.

Please do your own research to see if you'd like to try MCT powder:

Here is an explanation of "keto-flu": https://www.health.harvard.edu/blog/what-is-keto-flu-2018101815052

* MCT stands for Medium Chain Triglycerides. It's a healthy type of fat, usually extracted from coconut oil, sometimes from palm oil.

And here is some information about using MCT powders: https://uk.iherb.com/blog/mct-oil-keto-diet-benefits/1204

I have no affiliation with this company, but this is where I source my MCT oil. I do know the owner and I know that he is very conscious of sourcing quality, sustainable ingredients. https://shop.ketosource.co.uk/products/pure-c8-mct-powder

According to some experts MCT powder is more easily absorbed and has a greater effect on cognition. This trial by Dr. Stephen Cunnane used MCT powder: https://www.researchgate.net/publication/356286174_A_ketogenic_supplement_improves_white_matter_energy_supply_and_processing_speed_in_mild_cognitive_impairment

Case Study:

A client of mine who said she, "never eats any vegetables" and "fats make me feel queasy", but who wanted to implement the Bredesen Protocol® and as part of that, do the Keto Flex 12/3 diet, initially thought she would struggle because of her dislike of vegetables and fats.

On further enquiry, it turned out that she did eat some vegetables: onions, for example and she enjoyed soups; she could also manage olive oil. It transpired that it was mainly cheap fats, trans-fats, greasy take-away food that was the problem fat-wise.

Whilst she definitely said she would, "try anything", anything I suggested was met with a look of distaste. So, we started by looking at what she was already eating. She liked to eat meat and fish and carbs like potatoes, rice and pasta.

I suggested trying to swap rice for cauliflower rice. She immediately said she didn't like cauliflower. However, we had a real breakthrough when she was given cauliflower rice at a meal cooked by her daughter. She loved it.

After that, my client was much more open-minded when I would ask, "what is it about x that you don't like?" Depending on whether it was taste or texture, we'd work out together how to add delicious flavours (herbs or spices) or to cook it differently to achieve a different texture.

What would you need to consider on starting a new diet? What are your food go-to's? What symbolism or celebrations are closely tied up to food for you? How will you find ways around these?

A word of warning:

Every client I have who starts the KetoFLEX 12/3™ diet, finds they have more energy, feels sharper mentally and really enjoys the diet... except one...

A client of mine tried MCT powder and had a really bad reaction to it. He was fatigued and confused but was determined to do the KetoFLEX 12/3™ diet. He started the diet and again had the same reaction - fatigue and confusion. For the first few days, he assumed it was "keto-flu", but it continued.

It turned out that one of his causes of cognitive decline was mould exposure. In a very few cases, people with toxins such as mould, Lyme disease or mercury exposure may find that the Keto diet is not the right way forward for them.

As with all diets, you should consult a doctor or nutritionist first. If you are concerned that you may have been exposed to mould, Lyme disease or mercury, do consult with a specialist first. You can find a Re:CODE™ 2.0 Practitioner here: https://www.apollohealthco.com/practitioner-locator/

or a Shoemaker Protocol Practitioner here: https://www.survivingmold.com/shoemaker-protocol/list-of-certified-practitioners

Emotional eating and snacks

Do you eat when you're bored? Lonely? Anxious? Or some other emotion?

....

....

The old adage, "if the problem isn't hunger, the answer isn't food" is true.

Try this 3-step process:

1. Spot the trigger. How will you notice the feeling before you reach for the snack?
2. Stop, take a pause, count down from 5, 4, 3, 2, 1 and ask yourself how are you actually feeling? What is the problem? What's causing this feeling?
3. What one small positive step can I take to (even partially) overcome it?

How will you remember to apply this?

....

....

You might want to apply the Tiny Habits® tools to this (as discussed in Chapter 3).

Or do you eat as a treat or a reward for "being good" or having "had a hard day"?

What other things do you enjoy that you could replace as your treat?

For example, a long, relaxing soak in the bath or meeting/phoning a friend for a catch-up

What else can you think of?

....

....

....

....

And if you do really need a snack, keto-friendly snacks include:

- Crudités and dips (eg: hummus)
- Boiled eggs
- Nuts and seeds

What else can you think of?

....

....

....

....

A word about your microbiome

What do you know about your microbiome (gut bugs)?

....

....

....

....

We all have bacteria living in our gut, that help us to digest food and absorb or create nutrients. Having the broadest range of healthy bacteria is very good for our health. Sometimes our bacteria can become out of balance, or we can lose some of the variety, particularly if we've been on antibiotics (repeatedly). Antibiotics don't just kill the bad bacteria; they also wipe out the good guys.

There are some things you can do to promote a healthy microbiome.

Pro-biotics are foods that have good bacteria in them; think fermented foods like kefir (very easy to make yourself, try Mad Millie's kefir kit), kimchi, sauerkraut, miso, kombucha. As with all things, a wide range of these foods would be better than sticking with just one.

Pre-biotics are foods that feed the good bacteria and encourage their growth, these are all vegetables and fruits. The widest range of different veggies every day covering all the colours (white/ beige, yellow, orange, red, green, purple/blue/black) every day will have the greatest impact.

Why not create a chart with all the colours on to put on your fridge so that you can tick off each colour? I've put one in the bonus materials here; https://www.thecognitivehealthcoach.co.uk/ book-bonus-materials.

If you'd like to work on planning your diet, take a look at Coaching Session 5 on page 150 in appendix 2

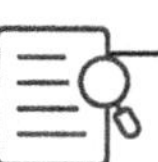

Case Study:

A client of mine was, in her own words, "not a great cook". She didn't enjoy standing, chopping and preparing food. Most of her meals were take-aways or frozen ready-meals. We started small, buying pre-chopped veggies and pre-prepared salads. Over time, she started to prepare some ingredients herself, and now she really enjoys cooking, she often shares recipes with me!

Here's another suggestion if I may; if you like the idea of making tiny changes, building up slowly over time, to embed them easily into your lifestyle, review chapter 4 including tiny habits and Coaching Session 4 on page 149

Reflection –
What are your key learning points from this chapter?

....

....

....

....

....

....

....

....

....

Chapter 6:
Moving

I've had a very up and down relationship with exercise in my life. I hated PE (physical education) at school, it seemed designed to make girls completely miserable! I didn't like the teachers, I didn't like getting hot and sweaty and I didn't like the shared showers. I hated running, I don't think I breathe properly, but no-one ever showed me how to breathe during running and PE teachers seemed completely unsympathetic to different children's needs or skills. When I think about exercise, this is what comes to mind.

However, I did enjoy some things as a kid, I enjoyed swimming, I liked tennis and in my early teens I started doing kung fu, I think the idea that it was something really different was appealing.

As I got a bit older, I found new things I enjoyed. I liked the social aspect of fitness classes like aerobics. In my early twenties I found skiing; I wish I'd learned to ski at a much younger age. I'd always loved dancing. It's funny how just the word exercise can bring such negative feelings, even though there are things that I did enjoy. Do you need to reframe any thoughts about exercise?

As I started a new job in my mid 30's as a trainer and coach, I found that I was travelling all over the country and indeed all over Europe and North America. It really disrupted my exercise again. I never felt I could start an exercise class, knowing that I'd miss more lessons than I could attend with all the travel for work. Looking back, I regret letting work get in the way of my health. Nevertheless, how many of us do exactly the same thing, putting work before our lives, families and fun? You're never going to find that on your death bed, your one regret is not putting in more hours in the office! Maybe it just takes getting a little older to get some perspective.

What activities did you enjoy as a child or young adult? What could you bring back?

In my 40's I had a herniated disc and I ended up having an operation to decompress it. The pain in the years running up to the operation and the stiffness afterwards really set my exercise back. After the operation, I found a Pilates teacher who focused on pain management and rehab and she helped me back to fitness. I was shocked at how weak I was at first. I had no idea how much muscle I must have lost, but it was clear from my difficulties in doing some of the exercises. The great news is that when we did repeat some of the same exercises after a while, it was clear how much I'd improved. I don't feel like I'm a natural athlete, nor do I feel like it's easy for me to put on muscle, but it was surprising how much more I was capable of in a fairly short space of time.

Even now, I start new exercise classes and I keep it up for months or even years, but something gets in the way, then I break the habit and it takes such a lot of work to get back into it. I also find that the getting ready and going is the worst part, I enjoy it when I get there, but it's easy for me to talk myself out of it: I've not got time, I've got so much to do. I really find that if I plan to do something with friends, I'm more likely to keep it up, for not wanting to let others down. What might help you?

Exercise is so important for brain health:

- It promotes good circulation, helping your brain to get the oxygen and nutrients it needs for top performance.
- One study[9] found cognitive decline is almost twice as common among adults who are inactive compared to those who are active
- According to neuroscientists[10] exercise decreases feelings of anxiety, improves focus and concentration, promotes the growth of new brain cells and protects the brain from aging and cognitive diseases.
- What's good for the heart is good for the brain, exercise also reduces inflammation and lowers stress levels.
- According to the Cleveland Clinic[11] exercising can increase the thickness of your cerebral cortex, improve integrity of the

white matter (the fibres that connect the nerve cells), promote neuroplasticity (helping your brain to change and grow) and improve your hippocampus (in charge of learning and memory)

Your self-assessment:

How often / how much do you move on average in a day?	
Do you get a good balance of strength (resistance), cardio (getting your heart rate up) and flexibility (stretching) training?	
What feelings come up when you are moving?	
What injuries or pains affect your movement?	
What things in your life do you prioritise, over movement?	
Add anything else you think of here	

As always, review your answers and make a note of anything that stands out to you, that you'd like to work on.

....

....

....

....

You might be interested in why I've entitled this chapter, "moving" rather than "exercise". Some people love to exercise, but for many people the word has quite negative associations either with school or the gym, for example.

Case Study:

A client of mine would shudder every time we talked about movement, never mind exercise! She associated it so strongly with some terrible PE class experiences at school. I noticed that when we talked more about what she'd enjoyed doing in the past (moving the conversation away from movement to hobbies and activities), it turned out that she'd loved clubbing; dancing the night away. We took some small steps to start with - dancing in the kitchen whilst cooking, teaching her husband to dance along to his favourite records (he'd never been one to get up on the dancefloor before). How much more enjoyable to include others in your hobbies and how much better for the brain, to include social interaction.

If you don't enjoy something, it's going to be very hard to build it into your lifestyle sustainably. So, if you fall into the camp of "not enjoying exercise", how could you find a different way of thinking about it?

Furthermore, different types of movement will suit different health types, even down to what time of day would be optimal for you. If, for example, you've worked really hard in the past, eating regularly, doing a strenuous "boot camp" first thing in the morning before work, stuck at it for months despite how exhausted it made you feel, and seen very little or no change in your body composition, chances are, this was not the right regime for your health type! The latest fads you find on the internet will work for some, but not everyone. It's time to start listening to your body. Your body is on your side. If you're working hard and seeing no change, maybe you're stressing your body with exercises that do not suit you. Find something you enjoy, remove the stress and watch things improve.

Movement could be really gentle, like tai chi or yoga, swimming or aqua aerobics, even walking counts and it's free!

If you'd like to work on planning movement, take a look at Coaching Session 6 on page 153 in appendix 2

Reflection –
What are your key learning points from this chapter?

....

....

....

....

....

....

....

....

....

Chapter 7:

Sleep

I really thought I was getting enough sleep. I usually got around 8 hours a night and I would find it quite easy to fall asleep at pretty much any time, so I didn't worry about going to bed at the same time every night. Apart from a period of stress I went through, my sleep seemed OK but I didn't really feel super refreshed in the mornings.

It was only when I got an Oura ring*, that I discovered I wasn't getting much REM or deep sleep. So, I started applying all the right sleep approaches:

- I made sure the bedroom was dark and cool,
- I started to go to bed at the same time every night,
- I tried a few evening Epsom salt baths,
- I stopped watching TV before sleeping in the bedroom, and instead started reading from my paperwhite kindle with quite a dark background setting (the paperwhite has a very matt, paper-like quality)
- I also got a lumie lamp alarm clock to wake me with bright light and a lumie lamp for my office for the darker winter mornings.

Now I'm really happy to report that my REM – Rapid Eye Movement (the stage of sleep when we're dreaming) and Deep sleep scores are greatly improved and I feel more alert in the mornings.

If you don't want to use a wearable device, here's a simple test you might try to test for sleep deprivation. It involves a test nap in bed in the day. Take a metal spoon with you and a tray. Get the room

* An Oura Ring is a wearable health tracking device. It measures heart rate, active and total calories burned, steps, sleep and stress in a lot of detail. Other devices are available. The Apple Watch, FitBit or Whoop have similar functions.

nice and dark and get comfy, dangle your arm out of the bed, holding the spoon outside of the bed with the tray underneath it. Take a look at the clock and note the time, close your eyes and relax. When you fall asleep you will drop the spoon and it'll land on the tray, waking you. Check the time. Proponents of this method say that if you fall asleep in less than 15 minutes, you may be a little sleep deprived.

Sleep is also very important for brain health. During sleep our brains:

- Store new information and memories
- Remove toxic waste
- Repair, restore energy, release hormones and proteins

You will recognise the feeling that on waking refreshed, you're more "switched on" but if you're particularly tired, your thinking can feel sluggish or foggy.

If you're struggling to sleep, or you feel that the quality of your sleep isn't good, you've probably tried a lot of things to improve it already. I can imagine that people have given you many tips for getting good sleep and I can empathise if it's frustrating that no-one really seems to understand quite what it's like.

Your self-assessment:

How many hours per night are you in bed on average?	
How many hours sleep do you get per night on average?	
Do you find it easy or hard to get to sleep?	
Do you wake in the night and struggle to get back to sleep?	
If you wake in the night, are you ruminating on the problems of the day? Or what else keeps you awake?	

If you are struggling to sleep, how long has this been going on?	
Are you taking any prescription or over-the-counter medications for sleep?	
Do you snore? Or do you sleep with your mouth open? Do you wake with a dry mouth or with a soggy pillow?	
If you wake in the night, what do you do then until you go back to sleep?	
What is your sleep routine? What do you do in the hours before bedtime?	
Is your room dark, quiet and cool at night?	
Do you use blue light screens (phones, tablets, etc.) before bed?	
Do you work shifts? If so, what are your coping mechanisms?	
Do you dream?	
Add anything else you think of here	

As always, review your answers and make a note of anything that stands out to you, that you'd like to work on.

....

....

....

....

If you'd like to work on sleep optimisation, take a look at Coaching Session 7 on page 157 in appendix 2

If you're the kind of person that loves to analyse data, maybe consider investing in something that can track your sleep; particularly if it will show your deep sleep (when your brain washes unwanted proteins out), REM sleep (when your hippocampus stores memories), light sleep and wakefulness. Look into an Oura Ring, Whoop, Apple Watch or FitBit® for example.

For more sleep tips, check out my YouTube channel: https://www.youtube.com/@thecognitivehealthcoach

For those of you with much more long-term sleep problems, if you've tried absolutely everything, then I have two recommendations.

1. This 8-part course is free and may give you some more ideas that you haven't yet tried: https://www.youtube.com/watch?v=lNdLGMVOS98

2. Once your insomnia has lasted for more than 3 months, there is a chance that you've reprogrammed your brain to a new (unhelpful) schedule. Cognitive Behavioural Therapy for Insomnia (CBTi) could help. This particular practitioner claims an 80% success rate:

https://sleepyheadclinic.co.uk/?msclkid=5f516dbaceb911ecb018f6041016acca

Reflection –
What are your key learning points from this chapter?

....

....

....

....

....

....

....

....

....

Chapter 8:

Stress

When my brain fog started, I was very stressed indeed, but if you'd asked me, I'd have said I wasn't stressed at all. Only now, looking back can I recognise how stressed I was. Stress is insidious, it grows slowly and we believe it's just "normal".

I was worried about my Mum's cognitive health. I was in the middle of trying to move Mum and Dad into a retirement village in the middle of a pandemic. My leadership development / executive coaching business had almost completely dried up, so my income had dried up too. I was waking up often at night worrying (I hadn't equated worry with stress!) and I thought I was handling it!

Acute stress on the mind or body can be really good for us. For example, a sauna, cold shower or going for a run are all great stressors that have a positive impact on our immune system and overall health.

Our bodies are designed to keep us safe, so our response to a stressful moment is "fight or flight", if we do fight or flee, we use up those stress hormones and that energy and we're soon back to normal. However, in today's world, often the stress just keeps piling up and we're never burning off that adrenaline or cortisol.

I definitely notice now if I start to struggle to find a word, if it happens a few times, I stop, think about what's changed and I usually find that I've become stressed again, without noticing, it's crept up on me.

How stressed are you? Are you aware of the things that trigger your stress? Do you notice the physiological changes that come with stress for you? How do you manage your stress?

....

....

....

....

I have to say that I'm not very good at meditating. That's quite an admission for a health coach! I am going to encourage you to try meditation. You don't have to be good at it; if you find your mind wanders a lot, you only need to notice it and let that thought go and return to whatever you were doing: counting breaths, body scanning, listening to a guided meditation, etc.

When I say I'm not good at it, I find I get quite stressed about it! My mind wanders and then I don't manage to calmly let the thought go. I stress over how much time I'm spending thinking about work or whatever. So, I've decided to relax in different ways. I like to sit and listen to music (quite often while I'm in the sauna). I've also re-found my joy in reading. I used to love to read and I could easily sit down and devour a book in one sitting. But as I was getting older, my eyesight was getting worse and I stopped reading. I'm glad I've started again now. Reading really transports me to another world, I get totally engrossed, to the point where I don't even hear if my husband speaks to me! I think that's as good as meditation. I'm totally focussed on one thing and not being distracted, nor ruminating on the same thoughts.

What activities do you do that you find get you into "flow", complete absorption, where time flies?

....

....

....

Breathing has also really helped me. When we take a deep breath (into our bellies, not a shallow breath where only our chest moves) and then breathe out more slowly than we breathed in, it massages our vagus nerve. The vagus nerve runs from our brain all the way down our body, past our diaphragm. It's a main communication route to and from the brain via the heart to the digestive system. When stimulated it triggers rest and digest mode. We can't be in rest and digest if we're in fight or flight. So, deep breathing actually massages the vagus nerve and can help us relax.

If you're not keen on meditating, could you just take a few long, slow, deep breaths either whenever you notice that things are getting on top of you, and/or at regular points during the day?

What trigger will you use to remember to breathe?

....

....

Your self-assessment:

How often do you notice negative self-talk? ("I'm such an idiot, I shouldn't have done that, why do I always"...etc.)	
Do you wake in the night and ruminate (think about things over and over)?	
How easy or difficult is it to balance all your work and life priorities?	
Do you have worries (financial, work, family, caring, etc.)?	
To what extent do you feel in control of the problems you face? (work, relationships, financial, etc.)	

Have you ever found yourself so stressed that you're "stuck", unable to move forward or to take in any new information?	
Do you find yourself catastrophising?... thinking through negative consequences to something that hasn't even happened yet.	
How often in a day do you just take a moment for yourself to breathe and to clear your mind?	
How often do you meditate or follow any mindfulness practices?	
How often in a day do you find yourself feeling grateful, or just appreciating something beautiful or excellent?	

If you'd like to work on stress management, take a look at Coaching Session 8 on page 160 in appendix 2

Here is an entertaining and very useful clip to watch, to help you start to find happiness and positivity in the small things: https://www.youtube.com/watch?v-GXy__kBVq1M&t-6s

I would encourage you to think more about contentment than happiness. Happiness is hard to maintain at all times. Everyone has mood changes. But if you can find contentment overall, that is a more attainable goal

And here's a great guided meditation app that actually learns from you and adapts to your needs: https://balanceapp.com/ msclkid= 5e16aa1fcf7511ecab69e61b175d1381

If you're still thinking about investing in an Oura Ring or an Apple watch, they also contain meditations and sleep guides.

Additionally, there is this free audio "brain entrainment" file that you could try that works on stress relief: https:// quantummindmethod.com

Reflection –
What are your key learning points from this chapter?

....

....

....

....

....

....

....

....

....

Chapter 9:
Stimulation

I've always loved learning. It's in my top character strengths. I have a very low threshold of boredom, so learning new things has been a way of life. When I'm facing a crisis, I turn to learning; I look at what I can learn to get me out of this hole!

When I first started work, I always enjoyed any training I could get and I always looked to sign up for any training courses available. After a few years in various jobs, I moved into training myself, then leadership development and executive coaching; I loved helping others to learn too.

On the break-up of a relationship in 1999 I turned to learning yet again. I started to learn to play the saxophone. I took lessons and eventually I joined a band. Music is great stimulation for the brain, so learning an instrument must be doubly beneficial!

Embarking on training as a Functional Medicine Health Coach and then the Apollo training as a Certified Re:CODE™ 2.0 Health Coach was a huge amount of learning. It suited me down to the ground. A lot of the training is quite medical, which I found fascinating! The ongoing CPD from both organisations keeps me busy.

Learning a language is great brain training. There is so much to learn. It can take years. I've been learning Italian for over 20 years on and off, (more off than on actually)! You'd think I'd have mastered it by now. I started around 1999/2000. I was working for Marconi Plc. at the time and they kindly paid for lessons with a native Italian speaker. I loved it. However, I left Marconi not long after and my Italian lessons fell by the wayside. I started again in around 2016 and I've been going to lessons on and off, working through textbooks with my husband, also on and off, but consistently using DuoLingo for the last couple of years.

It doesn't actually matter if you're getting really good at the language or if it's a constant struggle, because it's the challenge that strengthens your brain, not the success. Just make sure you're enjoying it. If you see it as a struggle, you won't want to keep it up. If you can look at it as all beneficial and just enjoy the process, it will do you good.

I also love listening to podcasts about functional medicine, about space, about the world and nature. I think a genuine curiosity about the world is a healthy thing.

What have you most enjoyed learning recently?

....

....

....

If you're not very focused on learning, you might not have noticed when you are learning something new. Reading this book is learning!

The old adage, "use it or lose it" applies as much to the brain as to any other muscle. There are studies showing that the more learning we have done in our lives, the lower our risk of dementia[12] It's called building Cognitive Reserve.

Learning stimulates new connections in the brain, stimulates the generation of new brain cells and builds up a functional reserve against future cell loss.

It's important to challenge your brain every day. You may well be a master at completing the New York Times Crossword, but if that's all you do every day to exercise your brain, then your brain gets used to working in this way; it's not being challenged to think in new ways.

Your self-assessment:

How often do you learn something new?	
How often do you feel really challenged?	
How much fun are you having with learning?	
How often do you feel really mentally tired at the end of the day?	
How often do you do things in a different way? (for example, taking a different route)	

If you'd like to work on brain stimulation, take a look at Coaching Session 9 on page 164 in appendix 2

Some new skills may take a long time to learn (e.g., a new language). Notice any self-talk when doing the new activities. If you notice any negative self-talk, try saying to yourself, "I'm not good at this... **yet**".

We all have a fixed mindset about some things and a growth mindset about others. An example of a fixed mindset is when you say something like, "I'm no good at maths" or "I'm just not creative", etc.

Think about a small child learning to walk. They fall many, many times. Never do you see them look up at you, thinking, "this walking thing, it's just not for me" and just give up. No, they keep trying until they have mastered it. They just assume that if you can do it, so can they. That's a great example of a growth mindset.

Very little comes "naturally" to anyone, but with practice and perseverance, you can master almost anything.

My own morning routine includes:

1. A game or two on BrainHQ. This app gives you different games to play every day, it learns what you're good at and will push you a little every time, then it pulls back just a little as you reach your maximum. There's a free version (1 game per day) but the very affordable license allows you to play more games and to tailor what you work on. If you're considering signing up with Apollo to do the Bredesen Protocol®, the BrainHQ subscription is included in their Re:CODE™ and Pre:CODE™ packages.
2. I do some DuoLingo; I've been learning Italian for many years, but it is a lifelong learning task! If I ever get to the point where I feel competent, I'll start a new language.
3. I play some games with friends and clients;
   - Wordle
   - Quordle
   - Worldle
   - Waffle
   - Blossom

...sharing our results on WhatsApp every day.

In addition, you might want to try this set of audio files on "brain entrainment" that work on stimulating your brain https://www.activemindsglobal.com/products/revita-mind/?wpam_id=1877

Case Study:

One person had a fantastic increase in cognitive scores through just adopting a ketogenic diet and doing BrainHQ https://v4.brainhq.com/?v4=true&fr=y for 30 minutes 5 times a week!

I love using my BrainHQ app. There are so many different games, it doesn't get boring. This is one of the only brain training games I've found that have real trial data to prove it works to improve your memory. The games start easy, but increase in difficulty until you start to fail, then they pull back a little. The next time that same game comes up in the future, it remembers your ability and starts just a little easier than what you achieved last time.

Reflection –
What are your key learning points from this chapter?

....

....

....

....

....

....

....

....

....

Chapter 10:

Detox

Before I found the Bredesen Protocol®, I always thought I was pretty healthy. I'd been mainly eating organic foods since the early 2000's, I'd never smoked, I felt that I was probably as healthy as pretty much anyone in the UK. Then I started to learn about all the chemicals present in other areas of our lives - plastics leaching chemicals into our food from bottles, wrappers and the lining of many tinned foods, aluminium foil wrapping our food, chemicals from cleaning products getting into our skin or breathing them in, non-stick pans leaching chemicals into our foods as we cook, never mind the chemicals they put in our personal care products.

I set out to detox my world. I replaced my plastic kettle with a stainless steel one. I stopped buying water in plastic bottles and bought a stainless-steel bottle to refill. I bought all new pans, which was expensive. It was one of the last things I did in my detox list, because of the expense, but I'm so glad I did it now. I bought a set of Tefal Ingenio Emotion stainless steel saucepans and titanium non-stick frying pans.

I mentioned in the food chapter that I use the Yuka app to scan all packaged foods and personal care products before I buy them to find the best products with no toxic chemicals.

Detox doesn't just apply to your food, but also to your whole environment and relationships!

Of course, our livers and our own body's inbuilt systems help us detox but just imagine how many more toxins we are exposed to in our modern world, compared to the world we were evolved to cope with.

Think about all the ways that toxins could make their way into our bodies:

1. Through the air we breathe,
2. In everything we eat,
3. From anything we put on our skin

Think about how many artificial products we use on ourselves or around our homes every day, never mind any toxins we might have been exposed to at work.

Case study:

One of my first clients started the Bredesen Protocol® with me and had some success in the early months, but then his progress really seemed to plateau. After extensive testing we discovered that he had heavy metal toxins from his work many years before as an engineer. Clearing these toxins was a longer process. First, we had to make sure his gut was in tip top condition, so that he'd be able to eliminate any toxins that were released, only then could we start supplementation to release, bind and eliminate the toxins.

A word of warning:

If you have been exposed to toxins, it can be very dangerous to release those toxins if you're not in a healthy place to be able to eliminate them.

Do contact a Re:CODE™ Practitioner here: https://www.apollohealthco.com/practitioner-locator/

or a Shoemaker Protocol Practitioner here: https://www.survivingmold.com/shoemaker-protocol/list-of-certified-practitioners if you're at all concerned that you may have been exposed to toxins.

Detoxing needs to be a long slow process. You should feel healthier during the detox, not worse. If you've ever tried to detox and found yourself feeling worse than ever, it is imperative that you approach it in the right way this time.

Your self-assessment:

How often do you use non-organic skin care products, cosmetics and perfume?	
How often do you use home care cleaning products that have a strong smell or are perfumed (e.g., lemon scented)?	
Do you use non-stick pans? (ceramic or titanium excluded)	
Have you been in contact with any toxic substances at work (now or in the past)?	
Do you go to the loo every day?	
Do you sweat freely most days?	
Are you involved in toxic relationships at home or work?*	
Are you taking long journeys in traffic (driving, taxi or cycling/ walking)? ie exposed to traffic fumes	
Is there any sign of mould or damp at home or at work (now or in the past)?	
Do you eat fish more than 3 times a week, especially large, top of the food chain, fish (eg tuna, swordfish, etc.)	

Do you have mercury amalgam fillings?	
Have you had a new car in the last 18 months? (new car smell is toxic)	
Have you had new soft furnishings, mattresses or carpets in the last 3 years? (soft furnishing "off-gas" for up to 18 months)	
How much water do you drink each day?	
Add anything else you think of here	

As always, review your answers and make a note of anything that stands out to you, that you'd like to work on.

If you'd like to work on detoxing take a look at Coaching Session 10 on page 166 in appendix 2

Here's another tip if you're interested. Did you know that houseplants "soak up" toxins in the atmosphere? There are even some that soak up mould (English Ivy is apparently the best for that) Check out the best house plants here: https://www.countryliving.com/uk/wellbeing/a668/houseplants-to-purify-house-air/

* Toxic relationships can have the same effect on our health as other toxins. Negative emotions and feelings of helplessness and hopelessness can create chronic stress, which upsets the body's hormone balance, depletes the brain chemicals required for happiness and damages the immune system. Chronic stress can actually decrease our lifespan

And a final word of advice on the topic:

If you are worried that there are toxins stored away in your body, it's really important to address these carefully. It could be more harmful to release these toxins into the body, if they end up circulating and not being eliminated.

It's important to know that your detox pathways are working well. Consider genetic testing to establish if you have good detox pathways, consider testing with an Apollo Practitioner or Functional Medicine practitioner to establish your toxic load. They will be able to advise you on a detox protocol to ensure that any toxins released are bound and eliminated, without causing you more problems.

Reflection –
What are your key learning points from this chapter?

....

....

....

....

....

....

....

....

....

Chapter 11:

Recreation / Fun

I've been guilty of focusing on work to the exclusion of life balance. I have a preoccupation with maintaining income and independence. However, I know, many years from now, on my deathbed, I won't be thinking, "I wish I'd spent more time in the office."

This is an ongoing struggle for me, particularly in peri-menopause, as I'm busy all day and then quite fatigued at night, though I do know that if I go out on a Friday night, the weekend feels so much longer.

Writing this book is also having an impact on time for fun. I spend most Saturday mornings writing, and that just puts back all the other things that need to be done before I can have fun.

Going out, seeing others, having fun is great for the brain in itself. The social interaction required might not seem like it's much, but think about what is happening in your brain... Just talking to others means listening, interpreting the words and the body language, it fires memories and connections in the brain to bring forth new ideas and contribute to the conversation. It's quite a workout! In addition, you're likely to get more exercise as part of the fun, so it's a double-whammy!

When I was younger, I loved art. I was always drawing or painting. When I started work, that all fell by the wayside. Now I've started going to some painting lessons and I'm really enjoying learning some new techniques and just throwing myself into a new hobby. I even went to a "painting with coffee" lesson – that means painting using coffee as paint, not having a coffee while I painted!

Here's my list of things to keep me busy when I retire. We're only at the planning stage at the moment and I have a lot more to achieve in my health coaching business yet, but still, it doesn't hurt to plan:

Days

Cycling

Exercise classes

Walking

Volunteering? National Trust?

Allotment

Evenings

Join a choir

Amateur dramatics

Book club

Holidays

Classes

Italian/ other language

Pottery

Art

Saxophone

Dance

Clubs

Astronomy club

U3A – University of the 3rd Age is a global organisation of local groups providing learning and social opportunities for retired people

Rainy days

Genealogy

...and, I am challenging myself to start as many of these as I can even before retirement.

What would be on your list?

....

....

....

Children spend a lot of time just having fun or even bringing fun to everyday activities. At what age do we "grow up"? And does that mean we lose our sense of fun? Think of the times when you've brought fun to an everyday activity: a work meeting, a brainstorming session or maybe had a work meeting outdoors for example. Were you more productive as a result? Are you (have you been) just too busy and got out of the habit? Or maybe you still find joy in the simple things in life:

Your self-assessment:

What do you do for fun?	
How often do you experience joy, laughter and pleasure?	
What did you used to do when you were younger, for fun?	
How long has it been since you partook of these activities?	
What would it be like to renew your interest in some of these activities, even if on a smaller scale?	
How do you bring fun to day-to-day activities? (e.g. walking outside meetings instead of in the office etc.)	

Add anything else you think of here	

As always, review your answers and make a note of anything that stands out to you, that you'd like to work on.

If you'd like to work on fun and recreation, take a look at Coaching Session 11 on page 169 in appendix 2.

Reflection –
What are your key learning points from this chapter?

....

....

....

....

....

....

....

....

....

Chapter 12:

Relationships (family and friends)

The older I am, it seems like the less time I spend with friends. Everyone is busy with families and work but I'm trying to prioritise friends and going out. I don't want to put off fun until I'm retired and have more time, but I do have quite a list of things to do when I do finally retire!

I've put some particular effort into making sure I see friends pretty regularly and so I usually set the next date at the end of any meet-up. I've also prioritised just a little time in my calendar, once a month to looking for new things to do: theatre plays to see, bands to see, activities to do. I've subscribed to local theatres, gig venues and cinema email lists, again to be prompted regularly.

What are some of your fun activities?

....

....

....

I am the kind of person who invests heavily in friendships. I have few friends but they are true friends; people I would drop everything for, to help in a crisis.

I have, in my life, culled a couple of friendships that were quite toxic. I probably took too long to do that, and I was affected by toxic comments. It's hard to specifically cut off a "friendship", particularly if you have mutual friends. I've struggled with cutting off relationships in my life, always trying to "see the best" or "give the benefit of the doubt", but I have no doubt that it's not been good for my view of myself and self-talk.

Contrary to this, I have noticed that quite a few of my clients have similar personality traits, quite the opposite of me. They are quite introverted and hyper-vigilant, noticing slights and perceiving negativity where potentially there only exists misunderstanding, cutting off friendships easily.

Case Study:

A client of mine was struggling with getting out enough and getting stimulation. She had withdrawn from quite a few groups, because one person there had said something that made her uncomfortable or had tried to engage her in gossip.

After some discussion, she decided to reacquaint herself with these groups, but to be more selective in where to sit, who she engages with and how much she engages. Now if some gossip starts, she can easily move away to chat to others.

We also role-played some situations to find a comfortable way for her, in one-to-one situations to gently let the other person know that she didn't want to get involved in a particular topic or to move the topic on lightly to something less problematic.

The impact of toxic relationships on brain health

According to Charlie Health[13], *"Toxic relationships can have a significant impact on an individual's mental health. The harmful behaviour in a toxic relationship, such as criticism, belittling, manipulation, and control, can cause emotional distress, leading to mental health problems such as anxiety, depression, and low self-esteem."*

Furthermore, a study in the National Library of Medicine[14], *"suggests an association between depression and dementia, … earlier-life depression or depressive symptoms consistently have been shown to be associated with a two-fold or greater increase in risk of dementia. In summary, there is an association between midlife anxiety, depression and the onset of dementia."*

If you'd like to work on improving your relationships, take a look at Coaching Session 12 on page 171 in appendix 2.

Reflection –
What are your key learning points from this chapter?

....

....

....

....

....

....

....

....

....

Chapter 13:

Oral Health

Oral health is really important to brain health. I'd always taken it seriously (I thought) I always went to the NHS dentist and hygienist every six months. I'd never had any problems particularly. I did have one filling, that I'd had for so long, that I didn't even remember that it was there, until it got a bit wobbly and I ended up having it replaced not once, but 3 times! All mercury amalgam fillings, all drilled out with no protection for me against the drilled particles being swallowed or breathed in.

Later, the same filling was giving me problems, but by now I knew about the dangers of mercury amalgam fillings. I went to a private dentist. I had root canal work. This time, the dentist used a blue stretchy shield over the tooth to make sure that no mercury could end up in my mouth. By this time, I was seeing my Functional Medicine Practitioner and she gave me activated charcoal and chlorella to bind and eliminate any mercury that I breathed in.

I also had two other cracks filled, this time with white ceramic fillings, so now I'm mercury free!

I've since found a few Biological Dentists in the UK who practice SMART – Safe Mercury Amalgam Removal Technique. This involves the blue shield, but also breathing through a nose mask to stop any breathing in of the tiny mercury particles, plus wearing an apron to stop any going on your clothes and also using a strong extractor fan.

Find your own SMART dentist here:
https://iaomt.org/resources/safe-removal-amalgam-fillings/

According to some studies, p.gingivalis (the gingivitis/bleeding gums bug) has been found on autopsy in the brains of people with Alzheimer's Disease[15].

However, it's not just bleeding gums that can be a problem. Breathing through your mouth[16], the need for root canal work and mercury in our fillings[17] can all have an impact.

Nose breathing

1. When we breathe through our nose, the air is warmed and filtered through hairs, unlike when you breathe through your mouth.
2. Breathing through your nose releases nitric oxide, which expands blood vessels, allowing more nutrients and oxygen to be delivered to the brain[18].
3. Breathing through your mouth dries your mouth, allowing bad bacteria to take hold.

I genuinely did not think that I was breathing through my mouth during sleep, I don't wake with a dry mouth, nor a soggy pillow. But I tried mouth taping at night anyway, just to see if it might make any difference. If you're at all concerned, you could try that.

Case Study:

A client of mine was applying the Bredesen Protocol® thoroughly, but seeing little to no improvement... until I discovered that he was mouth breathing at night. He immediately started taping his mouth at night, which improved his sleep straight away.

Gum Disease

A new study by researchers at the University of Central Lancashire (UCLan)'s School of Dentistry[19] *has revealed that Alzheimer's disease may potentially be spread from infected teeth. "This study is the first to link both of these oral diseases with Alzheimer's disease via amyloid-beta protein, and if anyone notices that they're suffering from symptoms such as bleeding gums, bad breath, loose teeth, gum swellings or toothache, they should seek help from their dental team as soon as possible. Early diagnosis is vital, as successful treatment and management of these oral health issues are a key part of protecting your long-term brain and general health."*

Mercury Amalgam Fillings

A study in the National Library of Medicine[17] investigated the association between dental amalgam fillings and Alzheimer's Disease using large-scale data. The study results show that women exposed to mercury amalgam fillings were 1.132 times more likely to have Alzheimer's disease than were their non-exposed counterparts.

What are your daily oral health routines?

am	
pm	

What else are you aware of that you're not trying right now?

....

....

....

Do your gums bleed?	
Do you have mercury amalgam fillings? - What condition are they in?	

Do you need root canal work?	
Do you breathe through your mouth? - Even at night? (do you wake with a dry mouth or with a soggy pillow?)	
Do you visit a biological dentist?	
Do you visit the hygienist regularly?	
Do you brush twice a day for 2 minutes?	
Do you use an electric / sonic toothbrush?	
Do you floss?	
Do you use interdental (e.g. tepee) brushes?	
Do you oil-pull?	

More information on oil pulling overleaf

Anxiety around dental treatment

Some people are really anxious about visiting the dentist. Many dentists are now much more attuned to people's anxieties and provide a supportive environment and longer appointments, to allow for breaks to allow you time to calm.

I recognise that for some, this can be really distressing. What support do you feel you need to be able to visit the dentist?

For example, do you need a trusted friend to be with you? Would you prefer to be anaesthetised? Would some calming music, meditation or hypnotherapy help?

What else could you think of?

....

....

....

....

Oil Pulling

Oil pulling is a process of swishing coconut oil around your mouth, a little like using a mouth wash.

Whilst many studies show benefits on oral microbiome of oil pulling, recently some commentators[20] have suggested a negative effect of oil pulling if you have mercury amalgam fillings, as oil is intended to pull toxins from the mouth, there is some concern that it could pull mercury from fillings, releasing it into your mouth, so consider carefully before you make a decision to oil pull.

Buteyko Breathing

If you find that you're mouth breathing at night (or any time), you could try a course of Buteyko breathing. Find out more here: https://www.youtube.com/watch?v=mBqGS-vEIso

Try a test first, breathe normally for a few breaths, then on an out-breath, hold your breath. Count the seconds. Breathe back in as soon as you feel you need to. Don't hold your breath too long. You shouldn't start breathing with a desperate deep in-breath, only hold your breath as long as it takes until you feel the urge to breathe. How long did you count for? .... seconds.

Whatever your count, you can increase this count with some practice, "breathing light". Breathe really softly, try to diminish the amount of air coming in, try to make almost no movements during breathing.

Practice this every day for a week, then try the test again. .... seconds. Did you increase your count?

Buteyko breathing includes many more techniques to help you

breathe more freely, clear congestion and nose breathe more naturally.

Removal of Mercury Amalgam Fillings

If you're worried about your fillings, first, get a toxin test from an Apollo Practitioner or Functional Medicine Practitioner. It would be a shame to take radical action before finding out if your fillings are stable or deteriorating.

Case Study:

Before I ever met her, a client of mine who had suffered terribly with toxins (mercury and mould) had all her teeth removed as she could see no other safe, affordable way to remove the large number of mercury amalgam fillings.

I wish I'd met her earlier, she could have had just the fillings removed, using the SMART approach I detailed earlier in this chapter

For more oral health tips, check out my YouTube Channel: https://www.youtube.com/@thecognitivehealthcoach

Reflection –
What are your key learning points from this chapter?

....

....

....

....

....

....

....

Chapter 14:

Finding meaning and purpose in life

This is such a poignant thing for me, I've always used work as my purpose. In the pandemic, when my training and leadership development business fell apart, I became depressed really quickly. I'd never really struggled with mental health before, so this came as quite a shock. In fact, I didn't even realise that I was depressed. I wasn't getting up in the mornings, when I did finally get up, sometimes I wasn't even getting showered or dressed, all day! It's obvious to me now that I was depressed, but at the time, I just thought there was nothing to do, so what was the point?

One funny thing is that after the pandemic, after I was feeling better, I asked my husband had he noticed that I was depressed? He had, but he just didn't know what to do about it. Who would notice if you were struggling? Who would challenge you?

....

....

....

When I finally determined to make a change and decided to lose some weight (I'd also been eating badly and drinking a little too much wine) and found the Bredesen Protocol® via a keto diet forum, I got so excited! Here was something I could do to help my Mum, and then not long after we started seeing some results, it gave me the purpose to train as a Re:CODE™ Health Coach and tell everyone that finally there is something that can be done.

But notice, my purpose is all about work again!

There are other things that are important to me in life. I've always loved to travel and my husband shares that joy. I have a goal to visit as many countries and experience as much of the variety of nature and different cultures in the world before I'm done.

We bought a "scratch-off map" to keep track of our progress as a bit of fun. Before we got it, I'd always considered myself well-travelled, but when we first started scratching off the countries we'd already visited, I realised that the world was a lot bigger than you'd think and that we have a lot more to do!

This is an-online version, where you can only tick off the whole country, so it looks a lot better than my real one where I've only scratched off a small part of China, Canada and Russia and where I've only counted the actual states we've been to in the US, so the outcome looks like I've travelled a lot more than my real map shows. But, either way, I would like to do more! The white countries are the ones I have yet to visit.

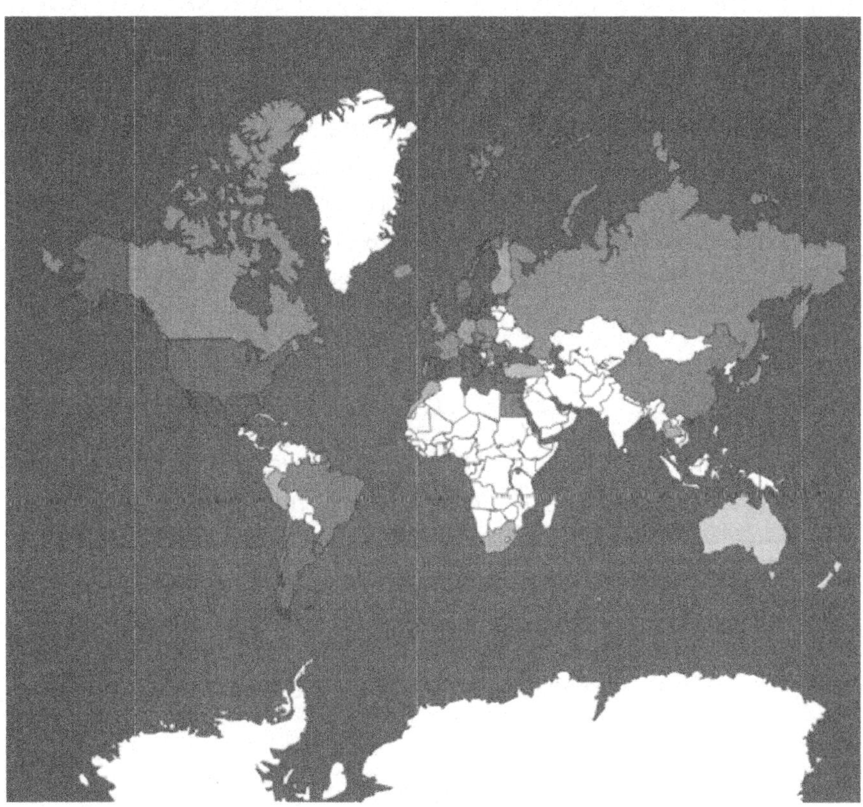

Have you ever heard of someone who beats an illness with positivity, or who, despite ill health, "hangs on" to see the birth of a grand-child, or the marriage of a child? It's amazing what that will-to-live can help us achieve.

If you've had a high-powered career, or a meaningful vocation in life, but felt a little lost on retirement, you'll recognise what we're talking about here.

It's not necessarily about achieving big things though, it could be about the small things that you do every day: Bringing a smile to someone's face, making the world a better, calmer place with your interactions, or just recognising beauty or excellence in the world, enjoying a beautiful day.

Maybe, you're still working. Are you letting work be your priority? That's fine, if that's what really motivates you. If it gives you the urge to keep healthy to keep contributing in the long term, great! Let me just challenge that though... What will you do when you do retire? Is it worth finding some meaning outside of work to balance it out?

If you'd like to work on finding meaning and purpose in life, take a look at Coaching Session 13 on page 178 in appendix 2.

Reflection –
What are your key learning points from this chapter?

....

....

....

....

....

....

....

....

....

Chapter 15:
Physical environment

Your physical environment takes into account everything around you, where you live in the world, where and how your home is, where you work.

My environment is very important to me, I find myself stressed if I am working in a mess or if the house is untidy, but once the house is thoroughly cleaned, I feel so much better about everything!

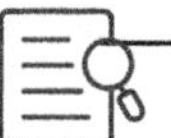

Case Study:

One of my clients was living in a real mess. She'd term it "clutter". She'd been experiencing cognitive issues for so long and been determinedly battling them, that she had no energy for housework or decluttering. Her husband was a rock, he was working full time, but did a lot around the house to help out too. But she was getting overwhelmed with just the idea of de-cluttering and every time she tried, she just ended up with more bags and boxes in more places all over the house!

I never thought I'd be coaching on interior design! But we took it one tiny step at a time, and instead of focusing on how much needed to be done, we talked about picking just one room and then thinking about what the purpose of that room was and what atmosphere it needed, to suit that purpose. We imagined the tiniest things that could be done to take a small step in that direction. That turned out to be a throw in the right colour and a vase for flowers; and one small step at a time she designed a room to relax in, to journal in and to find herself. (it doubled up as the grandkids room too).

The great thing about that room was that it gave her the energy to do some more, to move onto the next room, and before too long she felt totally "on top of it".

Your self-assessment:

Are you a bit like that? Is your environment getting you down or stopping you from achieving everything you might?

Where you live in the world: Does the climate suit you?	
What is the outside pollution like?	
What amenities do you enjoy / miss being "on your doorstep"	
Add anything else you can think of around your place in the world here	
Where do you live: How happy are you with your home space?	
How do you feel about your storage; tidy, cluttered?	
How comfortable is your furniture for your needs?	
Do you work from home? If so, is your workspace and furniture appropriate or is it causing you stress or discomfort?	
Do you / everyone in the household have a safe space to get away from it all?	
Where do you all come together for communal space? What activities do you do together? What do you wish you did together?	
Do you have outside space you can use to get close to nature?	
Add anything else you can think of around your home environment here	

Where do you work? How long is your commute?	
What are the ergonomics like at work? Are you comfortable?	
What are your relationships like at work?	
What stresses are placed on you at work?	
How do you enjoy your work?	
How does your work use your strengths and how does it challenge you?	
How does the temperature and ventilation suit you at work?	
Add anything else you can think of around your work environment here	

And now, what stands out to you in this assessment?

....

....

....

We might need to get quite creative in how to affect some of these areas! For example, if you feel that your work is not using your strengths or challenging you, you might not feel like now is a good time to change jobs or retrain for a new career. However, what could you do in the short term to get involved in some new areas at work that could stretch you (until you can make a longer-term decision about your career)? Who could help you in this endeavour?

Or perhaps where you live in the world right now is not suiting you, but it's not the right time to think about emigrating! What could you do to affect your climate in the short term (eg a SAD lamp) or to enjoy holidays in a better climate for you more often, to give yourself a regular boost?

If you'd like to work on your environment, take a look at Coaching Session 14 on page 184 in appendix 2.

Reflection –
What are your key learning points from this chapter?

....

....

....

....

....

....

....

....

....

Chapter 16:

Review and maintenance

Firstly, how are you getting on? Do you need a bit more support? Would you like to join my free FaceBook group here: https://www.facebook.com/groups/hopeinalzheimersuk

You'll find a community to help you with the little things plus lots of tips, resources, videos and recipes.

Review. Let's redo our original self-assessment.

Symptoms	Not at all	A little	Quite a bit	Extremely
Forgetfulness (e.g., walk into a room and forget why)				
Brain fog (e.g., lose train of thought, difficulty finding words)				
Difficulty focusing (e.g., read same paragraph many times)				
Difficulty learning new things, retaining information				
Difficulty adding up the bill, calculating tips etc.				
Handwriting has deteriorated				
Got lost driving (e.g., momentarily didn't recognise surroundings)				

Symptoms		Not at all	A little	Quite a bit	Extremely
Depression/lack of motivation (e.g., no longer find joy in hobbies)					
Poor sleep	Trouble getting to sleep				
	Waking in the night				
	Ruminating on thoughts in the night				
Quick to anger					
Slower movements or reactions					
Winter blues (SAD – seasonal affective disorder)					
Can't hear when there's background noise, or tinnitus					
Balance problems (e.g., feeling wobbly, must hold onto stair rail)					
Fatigued					
Flaky nails, white spots on nails, nail fungus					
Cold hands or feet / cramps					
Dry eyes					
Bladder control problems					
Reduced libido					
Bleeding gums					

Risks for poor cognitive health

	Yes	No
A family history of Alzheimer's Disease or another dementia		
Stubborn belly fat		
Brain trauma (accident or sports injury)		
Insulin resistance / pre-diabetes / type II diabetes		
Exposure to toxins or mould (e.g., at work, home or hobbies)		
Mercury amalgam fillings		

Compare it to your original results. How far have you come? What really stands out for you?

....

....

....

....

Have you retaken the cognitive assessment? https://www.apollohealthco.com/cognitive-assessment/

How do your new results compare?

....

....

....

....

....

Let's also redo the Wellness 360

Take some time to reflect on each topic, then please mark each spoke from 0 at the centre, to 10 at the rim of the wheel, then join the dots to create a plan as in this example:

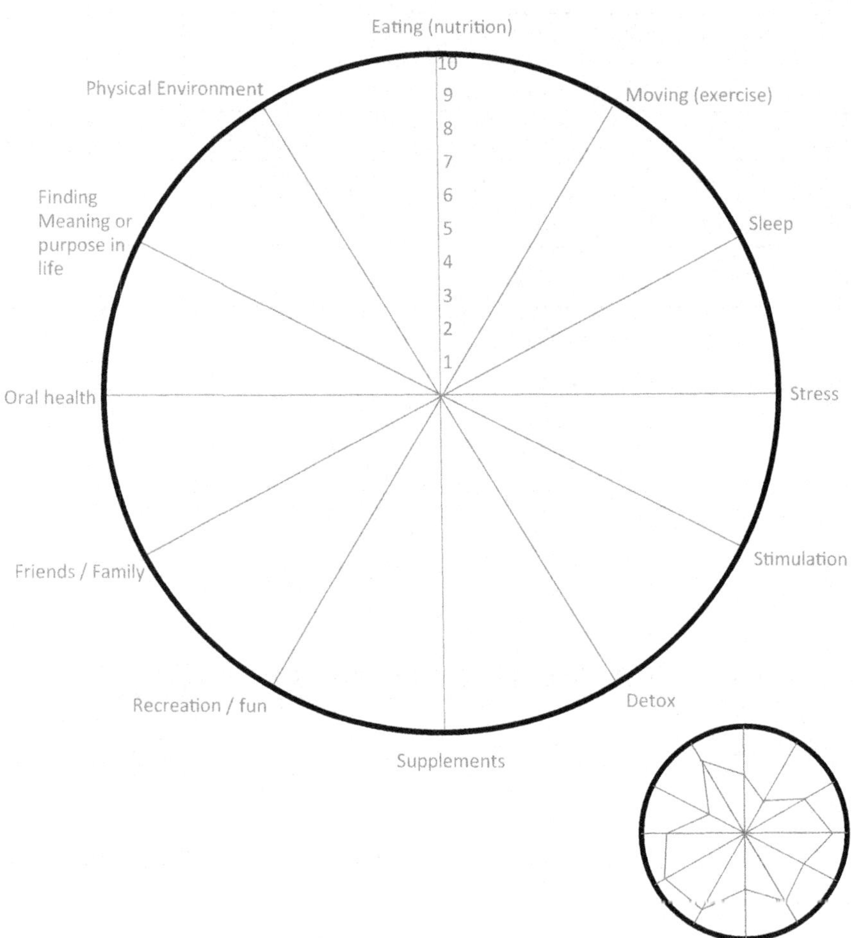

Compare this to your original map. How much difference has all your work made?

....

....

....

Let's just take some time to celebrate how much you have achieved. How will you celebrate?

....

....

....

Are there still areas that you'd like to work on to get even better results? Brain health is a journey, not a final destination! Go back to each chapter for each area you still want to improve even further. Work through the coaching activities again. Make a note of your new actions.

Would you benefit from getting some professional coaching support?

Is now the time to think about engaging an Apollo Practitioner or a Functional Medicine Practitioner to do more in depth testing to get some precision advice? You've come so far and made so many changes, any testing you choose to do now, any "prescription" for lifestyle change and/or supplements from a Practitioner is coming from where you are at your best possible healthy place through making your own changes. You're now working on the final tiny pieces of the puzzle.

However well you have implemented the suggestions in this book, you may still feel that you have more to do and you'd like some support. If you'd like to work with a health coach, here are some tips for you:

Health Coaching

So, what is the role of a health coach?

Have you ever visited your GP or MD and been told to eat more healthily and get more exercise? What exactly did they mean? What changes did they want you to prioritise? How did you implement these changes into your life in a sustainable, enjoyable way?

Unless you find ways to implement changes that you will enjoy, you are destined to fail, it's not your fault, it is human nature! And as Dr. Pat Williams, certified coach, says; "if you could have done it by yourself, you probably would have, by now!"

The role of a health coach is to stand beside you as a guide, not to tell you what to do as an expert. We are different from traditional doctors, but also different from Functional Medicine Practitioners too. Your practitioner is an expert in their field; a medical professional with additional training in functional medicine, they will recommend lifestyle changes and supplementation to heal the whole of you.

Your health coach will listen to you, really listen. There is no judgement, they will see you as a whole, intelligent, creative person. They will help you to find your own best solutions (alongside the recommendations from your Practitioner) to prioritise, implement and enjoy your new lifestyle. And where it's difficult they will help you to find workarounds or tiny changes to start the ball rolling.

Your health coach will help you to overcome the sense of "safety" that is holding you where you are now. Even in the midst of a health crisis, we can feel safe or comfortable, doing what we have always done. Your health coach will help you to face growth, no matter where you are right now, to take responsibility for your choices and make the changes you want to see in yourself. They can help you to examine your self-talk, peer norms and find ways to overcome whatever is holding you back.

Sometimes you might work with your health coach first, they will help you to write up a timeline to identify all the relevant factors; right from your mother's pregnancy and your birth, to today; identifying changes, traumas, lifestyle, stressors, relationships, changes in nutrition and movement that lead to the symptoms you're noticing now. Then your coach can advise your Practitioner of the pertinent points and help the Practitioner to determine what tests might be needed.

At other times, you might meet your coach after your Practitioner has made their recommendations and the coach will help you to implement.

Where you may have tried to make changes to your lifestyle

in the past and failed, they will stand beside you, help you find your motivation to start, and more importantly, your motivation to sustainably implement and enjoy your new life changes. Motivation changes over time and a strong desire to get started might not be enough to keep us going when things are difficult, when other areas of our life and relationships impact on our efforts.

If you decide to work with a health coach

If you're planning on working with a health coach, there are some things that you might want to consider to ensure you find someone you can work well with.

A colleague of mine from FMCA recommends asking these questions, thank you Eloise Bell FMCHC, for your wise words:

> *In a world where everyone is a 'life' or 'transformation' coach I thought it might be helpful to write some guidance to ensure that when you decide to go for coaching, you can be sure you have chosen someone of the highest quality that is qualified and regulated in case anything goes wrong.*
>
> *There are lots of stories in the press these days about fraud with internet-based coaches so I want to help you make the right choice to change your life!*
>
> *These are my top 5 things to think about when choosing a coach:*
>
> *Qualifications / certifications: to what level are they qualified to coach? Coaching is becoming more regulated but there are still many that don't have qualifications or certifications to a good standard. They've done a quick cheap online course and now they're qualified apparently. Look on a coach's website for their qualifications and check them out. A certified coach may be listed on their certification body's directory (for example they may be listed on the FMCA and UKHCA directories)*
>
> *Scope of practice / regulated: high quality coaches will follow a scope of practice or regulations of their certification/federation/ association. This outlines what the coach is qualified and insured to do. For example, my scope of practice advises that I am not qualified to diagnose or prescribe to my clients. I am not*

a doctor. Run from the hills from anyone that isn't qualified and doesn't have a scope of practice, they could do more harm than good. A good scope of practice ensures that someone 'stays in their lane' and is focussing on your benefit not proving their expertise.

Insurance; coaches should always, always have professional liability insurance that is aligned with their scope of practice and be happy to share that information with you.

Niche / specialism: what are you wanting to achieve? Can you find a coach who has lived through that experience? Does your coach say they can fix anyone's every problem? Look for someone that resonates with you, that you can be honest with as you know they've been through similar.

Personality: this is a huge one, you want someone you can be truly honest with and that you can trust. How can you find this out before you sign up? Good coaches will offer a free intro call, when you can chat things through and find out if you get on before you sign up. Social media is a great way to get to know coaches too!

I hope this is helpful for you - coaching can be the best investment you ever make so be sure to choose carefully!

Eloise Bell FMCHC

I would add to this, we are all unique individuals, you may not find your fit straight away, you may need to talk to a few coaches before you find your best fit, don't give up at the first hurdle. You wouldn't walk into a shoe shop, try on one pair, then finding that they don't fit, leave, saying to yourself, "shoes, they're not for me!", no, you'd keep trying until you found the right pair, it's the same with health coaches. Talk to a few and compare before you make your choice.

How might you work with a health coach?

Functional Medicine is all about looking at the whole person, looking for the root causes (rather than putting a sticking plaster over the symptoms) and getting your body's systems back into balance.

You will not be working on just your diet. You could have the healthiest diet on the planet, but if you get up every day to the alarm clock, dreading your day, hating your job, hating your boss, stressed, telling yourself you hate what you're doing, you will not be well! A great diet is not going to counteract everything else in your life that is out of balance and stress is only one example! What about your sleep, movement, relationships, sense of meaning and purpose in life?

All the lifestyle factors work together in harmony to produce a healthy life, or else one element out of balance can have an impact on the whole.

Here's a great quote from Functional Medicine Practitioner, Dr. Mark Hyman, "you can't exercise your way out of a bad diet..."

If you are working with a health coach, they will guide you, but it will be your vision of health, your goals and your action plans they'll help you to take responsibility for.

With every one of my clients, all our work together is bespoke; I would start by assessing their needs, goals, readiness and willingness to change, their motivation, inner gremlins holding them back and agree with them a route through our work.

Make some notes here of what you want to ask your potential health coach to make sure you've found the right fit for you:

....

....

....

....

....

....

Appendices

Appendix 1 - Food colour chart

Colours	Monday	Tuesday	Wednesday	Thursday	Friday	Saturday	Sunday
Green							
White/ beige							
Yellow							
Orange							
Red							
Blue/ black/ purple							

Appendix 2 - Coaching templates

Coaching Session 1 - Motivation

The Edge Model*:

The edge model describes what happens to us when faced with any change. Here are some definitions for you:

The Edge

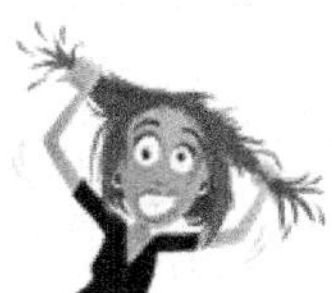

Your Primary:

A "comfortable" position that you find yourself in right now (through being tried and tested) no matter how unsatisfactory the primary may be, it is at least what you are used to.

Your Secondary:

The place you are trying to get to, what is trying to happen, but to get there, you have to get over your edge; that sticking point stopping you making the leap.

So, let's move into our first coaching activity, to see how we can use this model:

* reproduced by kind permission of CRR Global

The Edge

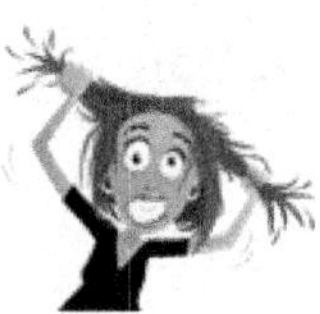

List all your reasons for staying in your primary:

eg; my friends and family aren't supportive of this change

…………………………………………………

…………………………………………………

…………………………………………………

…………………………………………………

…………………………………………………

…………………………………………………

…………………………………………………

…………………………………………………

…………………………………………………

…………………………………………………

…………………………………………………

List all your reasons for moving to your secondary

eg; I want to see my grandkids grow & have a relationship with them

…………………………………………………

…………………………………………………

…………………………………………………

…………………………………………………

…………………………………………………

…………………………………………………

…………………………………………………

…………………………………………………

…………………………………………………

…………………………………………………

…………………………………………………

Now, return to each list (primary and secondary) and give each item listed a weighting out of 5: where 1 is not very strong (in primary, not a strong reason to stay put and in secondary not a strong reason to move) and 5 is very strong.

Total up each column (primary and secondary)

Now return to each list and here, make a list of all the things you could do right now to make the primary list much weaker and the secondary list much stronger:

How could you minimise the primary?	How could you strengthen the secondary?
Eg: sit down and explain the importance to me and ask for help	Imagine attending their 18th/21st parties, graduations, weddings
....	....
....	....
....	....
....	....
....	....
....	....
....	....
....	....
....	....
....	....
....	....
....	....
....	....

How are you feeling right now?

....

....

....

What specifically has this inspired you to do?

....

....

....

....

When will you do it? How often? For how long?

....

....

....

....

What might get in the way?

....

....

....

....

How will you overcome these obstacles?

....

....

....

....

Coaching Session 2 – Keeping the Motivation:

Pick a realistic timeframe for this work. It could be six months, or a year, or more, depending on where you are right now and what you want to achieve.

Once you have picked that timeframe, come with me now, into the future, to the point in time you've picked. Stand with me in the future. You have achieved everything that you wanted to. We are "high-fiving" each other and celebrating your success.

Describe to me now how your life is:

- Where are you?
- Where are you standing?
- What are you doing (what are you able to do)?
- What are you wearing?
- Who are you with?
- What are they saying to you?
- What have been the benefits along the way?
- What are you able to do now that you couldn't before?
- What are you looking forward to?

Embellish this "future memory", feel how you feel, see what you will see, make it bigger and bolder and brighter:

....

....

....

....

....

....

....

....

It's important to keep this future you in mind. To phrase it in the positive, to give yourself something to work towards, to review and recall it often, to keep it alive.

Have you ever set yourself a goal, but found over time that your motivation waned? That you 'fell off the wagon'? Reflect on that goal for a moment. Was it a positive future goal, or a negative, 'get away from' goal?

People often make the mistake of phrasing their goal in the negative; in terms of what they want to get away from; what they want to stop. For example, 'I want to lose weight'. That might sound positive, but you're focusing on the negative thing, the weight.

Our brains struggle to process a negative, without thinking of the thing first. Whatever you do, don't think of pink elephants! What are you thinking of right now?

If you have (or have had) small children, think of one holding a glass of a dark red drink, full to the brim. If you say, "don't drop it!" what will happen? You've probably learned to say, "hold it tight" or "carry it carefully".

The problem with a goal focusing on the negative (ie weight) is, as you lose some weight, you are moving away from the problem (the weight) and as you start to lose weight, the push to continue gets weaker as you get further away from the problem; the weight.

If you focus on a future, positive you, 'I want to fit into my blue dress', then as you get closer and closer to it, the motivation is strengthening. The pull of the blue dress gets closer and stronger.

Take a moment to reflect on your goal from the coaching activity above. Is it future oriented? Is it positive? Make any adjustments you need to, now.

We'll come back to this aspiration a little later, we'll use it to set some longer-term goals and some shorter-term actions.

Coaching Session 3 – Character Strengths:

I'd recommend taking the test (it's free to register and you won't get unnecessary emails) at: https://www.viacharacter.org/survey/pro/lindseybyrne/account/register generating the report and then spending a little time considering:

How do you use the top 5-7 (signature) strengths in your life and career already?

....

....

....

....

....

....

How can you leverage these strengths to help you with the changes you're looking to make?

....

....

....

....

....

....

In order to familiarise yourself with your strengths and to leverage them in more situations:

a. Pick a different strength every week to focus on, to bring it forth in new situations

....

....

....

....

b. Start noticing (out loud) other people's strengths as they arise, and complimenting them on their use of their strengths.

....

....

....

....

c. Whenever things get difficult (whether that is with your current health journey, or more generally in your life or career) take a moment to take some breaths (to give you time to detach from the situation, to calm your stress response, and to break the drive to revert to old habits or behaviours) and then glance at your strengths report and pick which of your signature strengths you will bring forth to help you in this situation.

....

....

....

....

Coaching Session 4 - Creating Habits:

In his book, Tiny Habits, B J Fogg PhD, gives us much more information about what helps us to make behavioural changes, over and above simple motivation. New habits must be easy enough (or tiny enough) to overcome the need for great amounts of motivation. Motivation can wane, but if the habit is easy enough, you won't need motivation. We also need a prompt, or a trigger, something to remind us to do the new habit. A great prompt is to tack your new habit onto something that you're already doing habitually at roughly the time you'd like to start your new habit. E.g., "after I brush my teeth I will do ..... eg 1 stretch". Notice how tiny the habit is? 1 stretch! This is important. If you want it to be a habit, it needs to be SO easy to do, that nothing can get in the way.

Write your first one here:

After I, ...

I will ....

....

And now, how will you celebrate?

....

....

....

A simple, immediate "whoohoo" or other (silent if necessary?) celebration will programme your brain that this is a positive thing and you want to do it again and again. The small dopamine hit your brain gets when you celebrate a positive result is addictive; it's how you'll keep that habit up in future.

A word of advice: never increase your habit. Stick with the tiny habit, e.g. the 1 stretch. It's very likely that most days you'll carry on and do more but it's important to keep the habit tiny, so that even on the busiest days, there's no excuse to skip the habit.

Finally, return to the start of this coaching activity and do it again and again to make the next tiny changes.

Coaching Session 5 – Food plan:

You've made changes successfully in your life before, what character strengths did you use to achieve those changes? How did they help you? What specific strategies did you employ to stick at it and to overcome obstacles?

....

....

....

....

....

You might be a "get it done in one" kind of person or you might prefer to take small steps that are easy to fit into your lifestyle, one at a time, building on them over time. For example, rather than taking something out of your diet straight away and possibly feeling the restriction, what about adding something? Pick one thing that you can do to take one step towards a healthier diet and write below what exactly will you do, starting when, how often, how will you judge you have achieved it? Write a SMART objective below (Specific, measurable, achievable, relevant, time-bound)

....

....

....

....

....

What strengths (from session 3) will you be able to use to help with these changes?

....

....

....

....

....

Now let's take a look at what could get in the way? What obstacles can you foresee? And how will you overcome them? For example, do you have any parties or nights out coming up? What can you do to make better choices?

....

....

....

....

....

Who could support you in this, and how? Even if just to keep you accountable? Who could check in with you and make sure you're sticking to your plan? Or is there someone who could do it with you?

....

....

....

....

....

Thinking back to your overall, long-term goal, your vision for optimal health, that you described in Coaching Session 2, how does this small step move you towards your goal?

....

....

....

....

....

Once you have completed this task to your satisfaction, how will you celebrate?

....

....

....

....

....

Coaching Session 6 – Movement plan:

Look back over your life, what movement did you enjoy in the past? Maybe it was dancing, team games with school friends or with family, maybe it's swimming on holiday. Take a moment now to think back and make a list here of any movement that you've enjoyed in your life.

....

....

....

....

....

What was is about the activity that you found enjoyable (eg swimming on holiday, was it the warmth, the floating, the sights and smells)? Who were you with at the time?

....

....

....

....

....

What small thing could you do now to recreate a small part of that same feeling?

....

....

....

....

....

What planning or preparation do you need to do (eg get your bike serviced, find a local dance class, buy a swimming costume?) Who could support you in this?

....

....

....

....

....

What obstacles can you imagine getting in the way? How will you overcome them?

....

....

....

....

....

What strengths (from session 2) could help you?

....

....

....

....

....

Who can support you in this activity / how will you stay accountable?

....

....

....

....

....

What small changes could you make to get more movement into your life (park further away from the shops, take the stairs instead of the lift, etc.?) make a note of some ideas here:

....

....

....

....

....

Now that you have made some changes to your movement, perhaps you're feeling more energised, more confident and maybe you're ready to try some new activities. Why not get together with a friend or family member and do some brainstorming around some new activities that you'd like to try, here are a few ideas to get you started, add more in the space provided:

Cardio: Fitness classes: Aerobics Dancing	**Strength**: Pilates Gym training	**Resistance**: Press-ups, walking
Low impact: Swimming	**Flexibility and balance:** Yoga Tai chi	**Social / Team:** 5-a-side football Rambling club Tennis

Every time you find a way to build in more movement, how will you celebrate?

……………………………………………………………………………………

……………………………………………………………………………………

Once you have completed this task to your satisfaction, return to the start of this coaching activity and do it again and again to make the next tiny changes.

Coaching Session 7 – Sleep optimisation:

What are some of the things that you know about to help with sleep? Let's have a brainstorming session, I'll start (then you fill in some more ideas):

Take a bath before bed to relax and raise your temperature,

....

....

....

....

....

Which two of these would you like to try first?

....

....

....

How will you fit these into your life, how will you remember to do them?

....

....

....

....

....

How would it feel to start a sleep journal, recording what you've tried and how you slept, what works and how you've felt, to help keep you motivated?

……………………………………………………………………………………………………

……………………………………………………………………………………………………

……………………………………………………………………………………………………

Let's take a look at what could get in the way? What obstacles can you foresee? And how will you overcome them? For example, do you have any late nights out coming up? What can you do to balance this out?

……………………………………………………………………………………………………

……………………………………………………………………………………………………

……………………………………………………………………………………………………

……………………………………………………………………………………………………

……………………………………………………………………………………………………

Who could support you in this, and how? Even if just to keep you accountable? Who could check in with you and make sure you're sticking to your plan? Or is there someone who could do it with you?

……………………………………………………………………………………………………

……………………………………………………………………………………………………

……………………………………………………………………………………………………

……………………………………………………………………………………………………

……………………………………………………………………………………………………

Thinking back to your overall, long-term goal, your vision for optimal health, that you described in session 2, how does this small step move you towards your goal?

....

....

....

....

....

Once you have completed this task to your satisfaction, return to the start of this coaching activity and do it again and again to make the next tiny changes.

Finally, as you make each small change and you feel you've built it into a habit, how will you celebrate?

....

....

....

Coaching Session 8 - Stress Management:

Here are some simple things that you could try. Make a note against each that you think could help you, you might enjoy and that you would find easy to implement:

Activity	One to try?	What prompt or trigger will you use to remember to use it?
Guided meditation		
Take time out to breathe and clear your mind regularly throughout the day		
Reframe negative self-talk; challenge your own negative thinking, find a more positive way of looking at the situation		
Make an effort to notice positive things, beauty, excellence or the things you're grateful for		
Start a gratitude journal and write out 3, 5 or 10 things you're grateful for last thing at night before you go to sleep		

Make your first email of the day a positive one; thanking someone, or acknowledging a success		
Start (or increase) regular exercise		
Practice self-compassion. Whenever you talk to yourself, talk the way you would to a friend or small child		
Stop aiming for perfection, in any task, decide up front what will be "good enough".		
Separate your self-worth from your accomplishments. You are enough as you are		
Add any more ideas here		

Let's just pick one to start with: What will you actually do?

....

....

When will you do it? ....

....

For how long? ....

....

And how often?..

....

How will you know it's good enough (i.e. how will you measure success?)

....

....

Let's take a look at what could get in the way? What obstacles can you foresee? And how will you overcome them? For example, what will happen if someone wants you to do something for them when you'd scheduled a meditation? What choice will you make? How will you balance your needs vs the needs of others?

....

....

....

....

....

....

Who could support you in this, and how? Even if just to keep you accountable? Who could check in with you and make sure you're sticking to your plan? Or is there someone who could do it with you?

....

....

....

....

Thinking back to your overall, long-term goal, your vision for optimal health, that you described in Coaching Session 2, how does this small step move you towards your goal?

....

....

....

....

Once you have completed this task to your satisfaction, return to the start of this coaching activity and do it again and again to make the next tiny changes.

Finally, once you are completely happy with each new habit, how will you celebrate?

....

....

....

....

Coaching Session 9 – Brain stimulation:

Make a note here of all the things that you do regularly that are stimulating for the brain:

....

....

....

....

....

....

What do you notice about them? Are they quite similar, or are they very different? For example, if you love word puzzles, could you try a number puzzle? If you enjoy languages, could you try dancing, or music? Make a note here of all the activities you can think of that use very different skills, ie that use very different parts of the brain from the activities you already enjoy:

....

....

....

....

....

....

Who could help you start some of these activities? E.g., could you find a friend to join in?

....

....

....

....

Let's take a look at what could get in the way? What obstacles can you foresee? And how will you overcome them? For example, what if you feel tired at the time you'd scheduled to do one of these new activities? What will be your plan B?

....

....

....

....

And finally, thinking back to your overall, long-term goal, your vision for optimal health, that you described in Coaching Session 2, how does this small step move you towards your goal?

....

....

....

....

Once you have completed this task to your satisfaction, return to the start of this coaching activity and do it again and again to make the next tiny changes.

Finally, once you are completely happy with your new activities, how will you celebrate?

....

....

You might find with some of these new activities, that you're not very good at them at first. It's not important how good you are, just the learning in itself will be good for your brain.

Coaching Session 10 - Detox:

Referring back of all the toxins you identified in the self-assessment in chapter 9, what can you do to eliminate or minimise their effects? For example, what alternative products could you use, what alternative routes could you take, or how could you "clean up" your atmosphere?

....

....

....

....

....

....

....

....

Let's take a look at what could get in the way? What obstacles can you foresee? And how will you overcome them? For example, when you're in a rush and you're tempted to take the fast route? What can you do to make better choices?

....

....

....

....

....

....

If you're not currently going to the loo every day, how can you increase your fibre intake (plant-based foods, fresh veggies, fruit, nuts and seeds)? Make sure you start slowly and build up, else you may have an unwanted reaction!

....

....

....

....

....

....

What can you do to increase your intake of water every day to around 2 litres (start slowly and build up!)

....

....

....

....

....

....

How will you prompt yourself to remember to fetch more water? What would be a good trigger (e.g. every time you go to the bathroom, fetch some more water... don't forget to celebrate [whoohoo])

....

....

....

....

....

Who could support you in this, and how? Even if just to keep you accountable? Who could check in with you and make sure you're sticking to your plan? Or is there someone who could do it with you?

....

....

....

....

....

....

And finally, thinking back to your overall, long-term goal, your vision for optimal health, that you described in Coaching Session 2, how does this small step move you towards your goal?

....

....

....

....

....

....

Once you have completed this task to your satisfaction, return to the start of this coaching activity and do it again and again to make the next tiny changes.

Finally, once you are completely happy with how you are managing the toxins around you, how will you celebrate?

....

....

....

Coaching Session 11 – Fun and recreation:

Thinking of all the activities you identified in the previous self-assessment in chapter 10, which would you like to try out?

....

....

....

....

....

What do you need to research, plan, organise, arrange or buy up front to make this happen?

....

....

....

....

Who would you like to be involved?

....

....

....

Let's take a look at what could get in the way? What obstacles can you foresee? And how will you overcome them? For example, when you're in a rush and you're tempted to get things done quickly or to stick to your routine? What can you do to prioritise fun for yourself and others?

....

....

....

....

Who could support you in this, and how? Even if just to keep you accountable? Who could check in with you and make sure you're sticking to your plan? Or is there someone who could do it with you? Or even just brainstorm new ideas with?

....

....

....

....

....

And finally, thinking back to your overall, long-term goal, your vision for optimal health, that you described in Coaching Session 2, how does this small step move you towards your goal?

....

....

....

....

....

Return to the start of this coaching activity and do it again and again.

Remember to celebrate!

Coaching Session 12 – Relationships

We're going to create a "paper constellation"™* of the relationships you have with a group of people. It can be either for family, work or friends, or you can do this activity many times for every group you find yourself in.

First, using the space overleaf you will place yourself somewhere on the paper representing how "central" you feel to the group, using a circle if you're a woman or a triangle if you're a man.

Then place everyone else in the group (eg the family) on the paper too. If there is a specific event that you want to focus on, for example a Christmas lunch or a project, then that can be represented by a square.

Finally connect yourself with all the people and events shown with a line. Use either a single line if the relationship is OK, a dotted line if the relationship is poor or weak and a double line for a strong relationship. You can represent conflict in a relationship by a short double line crossing the linking line. Here's an example:

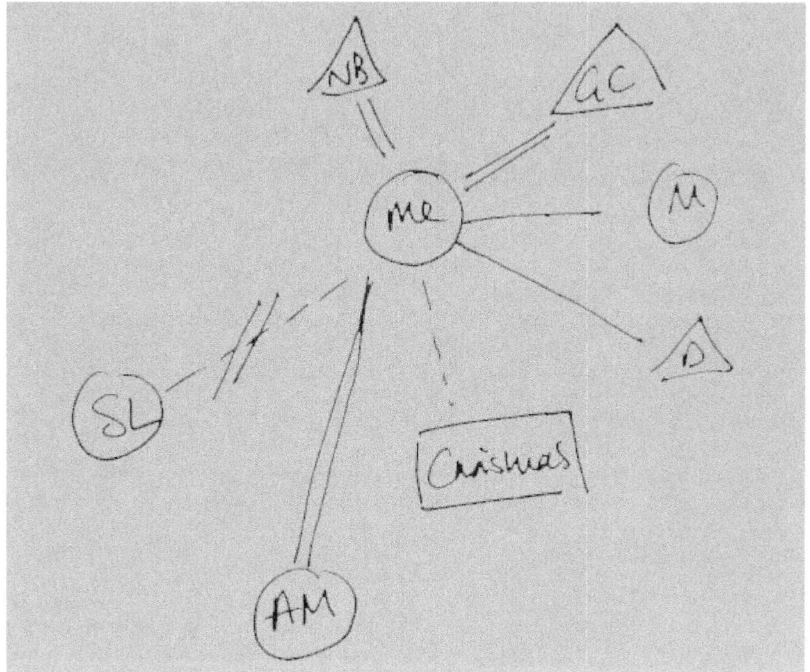

* Paper constellations from ORSC reproduced by kind permission of CRR Global

Key:

□	Event	———	Average relationship	//	Conflict
△	Man	·········	Poor relationship		
◯	Woman	═══	Strong relationship		

Now it's your turn:

What stands out to you from this constellation?

....

....

....

....

Now, create a new constellation, how you would like these relationships to be? Feel free to change the connectors, add or move players around.

Take a moment to "live" these new relationships. What would it feel like to have these relationships working this way? What are you doing together? What are you all saying? What is the atmosphere?

....

....

....

What is one small thing you can say or first step that you can do to move these relationships one step closer to this vision?

....

....

....

....

....

Working on relationships can be hard. It can feel uncomfortable to approach something that has been going on for a while and feels quite ingrained into the relationship. What could you say to open the conversation, that would feel comfortable to you to say? Actually 'say' these words out loud as if you're saying them to the other person now. How does it feel? Can you find a way to say them and feel comfortable with the words you're using?

....

....

....

Put yourself in the other person's shoes. We're going to do an activity to really try to see it from their point of view. Wherever you are right now, sitting or standing, move. Move to another point in the room, as if you were actually moving to stand in the other person's shoes in this conversation. It is actually really important that you do move. There is something special about movement that will really enhance this activity. Now, rehear your words you just spoke out loud, as if you were hearing them as the other person. What are their typical reactions and how might they react? Say their words as if you're saying them to yourself in conversation:

....

....

....

How did that feel to you to say those words? What insights have you gained? How did it feel to speak them? What insights have you gained from this interaction?

....

....

....

You may have gained a great deal of insight from this activity, or you may still be struggling.

a) It's absolutely fine if you don't know what they'd say or you don't get any insight into how they're feeling. That is information too! That's telling us that we need to get curious, to ask some questions, to find out where they're coming from. What do you want to ask them now?

....

....

....

b) If you did gain some insight from that interaction, what do you want to say to them now? Move back to the first position (where you were standing as you) to say it.

....

....

Feel free to move back and forth in the conversation between the two positions as much as you need to, to gain your insight.

Do you have a plan now? What exactly will you say to open the conversation?

....

....

....

What atmosphere would you like to bring to the conversation? E.g., calm, open, curious?

....

....

....

What tone, body language and words would embody that atmosphere?

....

....

....

What obstacles can you foresee, what might stop you? And how will you overcome them? For example, what if the time isn't right for them to get into this? What will you do then?

....

....

....

....

....

Who could support you in this, and how? Even if just to keep you accountable? Who could check in with you and make sure you're sticking to your plan?

....

....

....

....

Finally, thinking back to your overall, long-term goal, your vision for optimal health, that you described in Coaching Session 2, how does this small step move you towards your goal?

....

....

....

....

Once you have completed this task to your satisfaction, return to the start of this coaching activity and do it again and again to make the next tiny changes in the same relationship or in the next one.

Finally, once you have opened communications with each person, how will you celebrate?

....

....

....

....

Coaching Session 13 – Finding meaning and purpose

We're going to start straight out with an activity. Take a moment to imagine yourself in the future, looking back over your life, reviewing what you did, who you had an impact on, what your legacy for the world is. Ask yourself, how would you like people to remember you?

If you like, you could think of this as your eulogy.

It doesn't matter how big or small you feel your ambitions are. Any small positive things that you would like to do, to bring joy to yourself and others will be enough.

Don't worry about getting this "right", you could come back to this time and again, to add to it or hone it.

Reflect on what you've written. How do you feel now looking over this?

....

....

It might help you to think about what are your values; what is important to you in life? Take a look at this list and highlight all that stand out to you.

Then start to rank them. Find your top 5-10.

Acceptance	Accountability	Accuracy	Achievement
Adaptability	Advancement	Adventure	Agility
Altruism	Ambition	Approachability	Assertiveness
Awareness	Balance	Being the best	Belonging
Boldness	Calmness	Candour	Carefulness
Caring	Challenge	Charity	Cheerfulness
Clear-mindedness	Coaching/ mentoring	Comfort	Commitment
Community	Compassion	Competence	Competition
Conflict resolution	Conformity	Consistency	Contentment
Continuous improvement	Contribution	Control	Cooperation
Correctness	Courage	Courtesy	Creativity
Curiosity	Decisiveness	Democracy	Dependability
Determination	Devotion	Dialogue	Diligence
Discipline	Discretion	Diversity	Dynamism
Economy	Effectiveness	Efficacy	Efficiency
Elegance	Empathy	Enjoyment	Enthusiasm
Entrepreneurship	Environment	Equality	Ethics
Excellence	Excitement	Expertise	Exploration
Expressiveness	Fairness	Faith	Fame
Family	Fidelity	Financial stability	Fitness
Fluency	Focus	Forgiveness	Freedom
Friendship	Fun	Future generations	Generosity
Goodness	Grace	Growth	Happiness
Hard work	Health	Helping society	Holiness
Honesty	Honour	Humility	Humour
Impartiality	Independence	Ingenuity	Inner harmony

Inquisitiveness	Insightfulness	Integrity	Intelligence
Intellectual status	Intuition	Joy	Justice
Leadership	Learning	Legacy	Listening
Love	Loyalty	Making a difference	Mastery
Merit	Obedience	Openness	Order
Originality	Patience	Patriotism	Perfection
Perseverance	Philanthropy	Physical challenge	Piety
Positivity	Power	Practicality	Preparedness
Professionalism	Prudence	Public service	Quality-orientation
Recognition	Reliability	Reputation	Resourcefulness
Respect	Responsibility	Restraint	Results-orientation
Rigour	Risk taking	Security	Self-actualisation
Self-control	Self-discipline	Selflessness	Self-reliance
Sensitivity	Serenity	Service	Shrewdness
Simplicity	Soundness	Speed	Spontaneity
Stability	Status	Strength	Structure
Success	Support	Teamwork	Temperance
Thankfulness	Thoroughness	Thoughtfulness	Timeliness
Tolerance	Traditionalism	Trustworthiness	Truth-seeking
Understanding	Uniqueness	Unity	Usefulness
Vision	Vitality	Wealth	Wisdom
Now add any that are missing for you			

And now, which are your most important 5? (reduce your list from before if you had more than 5)

What do each mean to you? Take a moment to define each of your top 5 and think about the actions you take daily to live these values. What else could you do? What would leave you feeling satisfied that you are living your values?

Value	Definition	How do you/will you live them every day

Now go back to your "eulogy"; the first activity in this coaching session and consider and reflect on what you have learned from this values activity. What do you want to add to your eulogy now?

What small steps do you want to take in the next few weeks to live your values even better?

....

....

....

....

....

....

....

....

Let's take a look at what could get in the way. What obstacles can you foresee? And how will you overcome them?

....

....

....

....

....

....

....

....

Who could support you in this, and how? Even if just to keep you accountable? Who could check in with you and make sure you're sticking to your plan? Is there someone who could do it with you?

....

....

....

....

....

....

....

....

Thinking back to your overall, long-term goal, your vision for optimal health that you described in Coaching Session 2, how does this small step move you towards your goal?

....

....

....

....

....

....

....

....

Coaching Session 14 – Environment

Prioritise one achievable thing from the list in your self- assessment (page 128) that you want to work on. You can return to this activity at the end and repeat for each item, or you can return to it at a future date.

Take some time first of all, to imagine your perfect environment (in relation to this priority). Close your eyes. Really put yourself into this place; see what you would see, hear what you would hear, feel how you would feel. Who is with you? What is your day like in this place? Make the image bigger and bolder and brighter, really live it for a moment. Make some notes below:

....

....

....

....

....

Now take some time to examine some of the key things that really stood out for you in that image, what was it specifically about them that created good feelings?

....

....

....

....

....

Take each in turn. Is there a way of replicating those good feelings, even at the smallest level? Let's practice our brainstorming again. Thinking about recreating that feeling at a small level might mean taking one element, it might mean creating a small amount of time in your day to do something, it might mean taking a first step towards it:

....

....

....

....

....

Again, taking each in turn. What obstacles are presenting themselves? What can you do to overcome those obstacles? Who can help or support you?

....

....

....

....

And so now, what is your first step?

....

....

....

Who could support you in this, and how? Even if just to keep you accountable? Who could check in with you and make sure you're sticking to your plan? Or is there someone who could do it with you?

....

....

....

....

....

....

Thinking back to your overall, long-term goal, your vision for optimal health, that you described in Coaching Session 2, how does this small step move you towards your goal?

....

....

....

....

Once you have completed this task to your satisfaction, return to the start of this coaching activity and do it again and again to make the next tiny changes.

Finally, once you feel you are making steps to improve your environment, how will you celebrate?

....

....

Authors Bio

Lindsey specialises in using a Functional Medicine Health Coaching approach to help clients to:

- Prevent
- Slow the progression
- and even improve the symptoms of MCI (Mild Cognitive Impairment)

Lifestyle changes can be difficult to implement alone. No matter how motivated you are right now, this is a change for life, not a short-term fix.

She can help you to make small, step by step changes, prioritised specifically for you and your situation, to create long term, sustained improvements to your health and wellbeing, overcoming any obstacles you meet along the way and finding your own resources and strengths to flourish.

Health coaching is about understanding where you are right now, what your vision is for a future of optimum health, setting small, sustainable, realistic goals, prioritising the changes you want to make, providing resources where necessary, providing support and accountability to succeed.

See my listings here:
https://directory.functionalmedicinecoaching.org/england/coventry/health-coach/lindsey-byrne
and https://www.ukihca.com/england/coventry/health-coach/lindsey-byrne

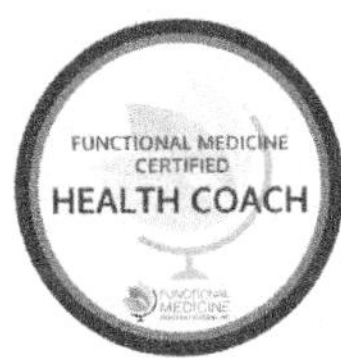

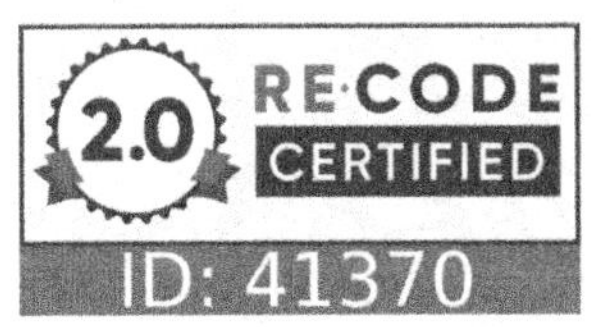

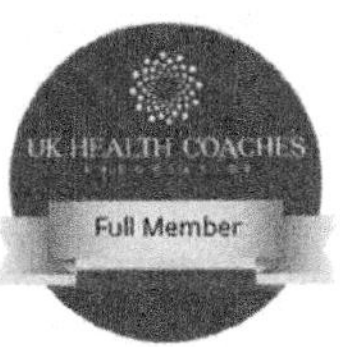

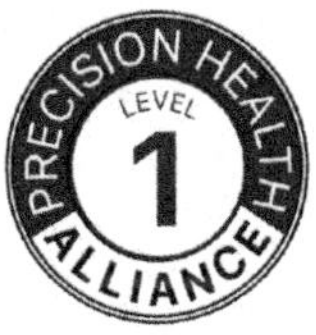

Acknowledgements

Any book on this subject will be the product of the author's exposure to and learning from many experiences with coaching clients, Re:CODE™ Practitioners, Functional Medicine (FM) Practitioners and Cognitive Health Professionals.

Particular thanks must go to:

My Mum, for giving this a go, despite the difficulties of age, poor mobility, difficulties with implementing the diet in her situation, but for sticking with the things she can do.

Jo Gamble of Embracing Nutrition for all her support with my Mum's cognitive health and my own early testing and dementia prevention strategies.

Dr. Michael Cannell for all his support with my clients: Bredesen testing panels, supplements and great advice.

The Functional Medicine Coaching Academy for their excellent training and ongoing support and continuing professional development.

The Institute of Functional Medicine for their research into the causes of chronic conditions, battling to get information out there that so many chronic conditions can be reversed through lifestyle change, for looking at the health of the whole person and working to balance all the systems in the body to optimise health.

Dr. Dale Bredesen and everyone at Apollo Health for pioneering research and developing and constantly honing protocols to help people regain their cognition. As well as all the excellent coach training and ongoing support and continuing professional development. Also for being so accessible to clients when they have specific questions, via the Apollo town hall meetings and social media. Rarely have I seen such a busy and high-profile figure, give so much time to those who need it.

Damien Blenkinsop and the Ketosource team for sharing research papers on the ketogenic diet and exogenous ketone supplements in the treatment of dementia.

James Kearns for bringing my attention to the world of FM and the possibilities for Alzheimer's reversal and for sharing his story so openly and generously.

My husband, Nick, for his continuing support in my health journey, both personal and professional and for all his help in reading, re-reading, editing and proofreading this book.

My friend, Dawn, for her amazing work proof-reading this, she did a thorough job when it's hard to spot your own errors. If this book reads well, it's all credit to Dawn. If you find mistakes or clunky phrases, the fault will be mine, I probably missed some of her suggestions.

My publisher, Clare, for all her support through this process, publishing a book is an arduous process, I couldn't have done it without her.

References

1. https://www.who.int
2. Benjamin C Trumble et al FASEB Journal 2017 https://faseb.onlinelibrary.wiley.com/doi/full/10.1096/fj.201601084R
3. The Alzheimer's Society https://www.alzheimers.org.uk/blog/how-much-does-dementia-care-cost
4. The Wheel of Life from Wellness Coaching for Lasting Lifestyle Change; Michael Arloski
5. The Wellness Workbook; Jack Travis & Regina Ryan 2004
6. The Bredesen 7; Apollo Health Co
7. Harvard school of public health - Friends, family can influence your weight – for good or bad.
8. Tiny Habits® by Prof B J Fogg
9. https://www.sciencedirect.com/science/article/abs/pii/S0091743520303030?via%3Dihub
10. https://www.cnbc.com/2021/10/22/neuroscientist-shares-the-brain-health-benefits-of-exercise-and-how-much-she-does-a-week.html
11. https://health.clevelandclinic.org/exercise-and-brain-health/
12. https://www.alzheimersresearchuk.org/differences-in-early-life-education-linked-to-dementia-risk/
13. https://www.charliehealth.com/post/how-toxic-relationships-affect-your-mental-health
14. https://www.ncbi.nlm.nih.gov/pmc/articles/PMC3327554/
15. https://pubmed.ncbi.nlm.nih.gov/30746447/

16. 16 https://jamanetwork.com/journals/jamaneurology/fullarticle/2763344
17. https://www.ncbi.nlm.nih.gov/pmc/articles/PMC4642684/
18. https://www.healthline.com/health/nose-breathing
19. https://www.dental-nursing.co.uk/news/research-directly-links-infected-teeth-and-alzheimers-disease
20. https://medium.com/@meliors/could-oil-pulling-put-you-at-risk-e9a428353a8c